Statistical Analysis in Primary Care

Edited by
Nigel Mathers
Martin Williams
and
Beverley Hancock

Foreword by
Mike Pringle

Radcliffe Medical Press

©2000 Trent Focus Group

Radcliffe Medical Press Ltd
18 Marcham Road, Abingdon, Oxon OX14 1AA

British Library Cataloguing in Publication Data

A catalogue record for this book is available from the British Library.

ISBN 1 85775 387 9

Typeset by Advance Typesetting Ltd, Oxfordshire
Printed and bound by TJ International Ltd, Padstow, Cornwall

Contents

Foreword

Research into primary care is underdeveloped, not just amongst general practitioners but also nurses and other health professionals. Primary care cannot be expected to move from the twilight into the spotlight without support. The welcome access for general practices and community trusts to Culyer research and development funding has started to redress the resource inequality between primary and secondary care. However, the greatest shortage has been in research skills, as those involved have not routinely been expected to undertake research in their training and, for many, research skills appear foreign and demanding.

The recognition of these realities led Trent Regional Health Authority – now the Trent Regional Office of the NHS Executive – to support the Trent Focus for the Promotion of Research and Development in Primary Health Care from 1995 onwards. The Focus has existed primarily to enhance the research skills of those working in primary care on a regional basis. It does this through offering education and support to those interested in research; buying specific research advice for those undertaking research; supporting research clubs; running a collaborating research practices scheme and funding designated research practices which undertake original research.

Out of this work recognition emerged that some research issues came up time and again, and that the standard reference works do not cover them satisfactorily. Thus the idea for this series was born. These volumes synthesise current wisdom on how to start successfully in primary care research. They are not intended to provide definitive texts, nor to be used as the only source of knowledge. They will, however, cover most of the issues that a nascent researcher will encounter, and will inspire many to try their hand.

For the truth is this: research can be wonderfully stimulating, enriching our daily clinical work and helping to improve care for future generations. However, like most areas of human activity, it is only worth doing if it is done well – and that requires skills, support, advice, insight and perseverance. Those who read and use these volumes will stand a better chance of doing good research, and should obtain real pleasure from it.

Professor Mike Pringle
Chairman
RCGP
October 1999

Volume editors

Professor Nigel Mathers
Director
Institute of General Practice
    and Primary Care
University of Sheffield

Martin Williams
Trent Focus Local Coordinator
De Montfort University

Beverley Hancock
Trent Focus Local Coordinator
Division of General Practice
University of Nottingham

List of contributors

Dr Kim Cornish
Postgraduate Division of Nursing and
    Division of Psychiatry
University of Nottingham

Dr Nick Fox
Institute of General Practice and
    Primary Care
University of Sheffield

Dr Michael Hewitt
Trent Institute for Health Services
    Research
University of Nottingham and
    Nottingham Community Health
    NHS Trust

Amanda Hunn
Trent Focus Local Coordinator
Institute of General Practice and
    Primary Care
University of Sheffield

Introduction

Nigel Mathers

Primary healthcare professionals often approach the subject of quantitative data analysis with a considerable degree of trepidation. It seems so difficult to many of us and, with only a few notable exceptions, the standard statistical tests seem dry and complicated. Most of our work time is spent looking after patients and there seems little time left over for research activity. It can be particularly difficult to find protected time to invest in learning new skills, such as statistical data analysis. Indeed many of us prefer to collect and analyse qualitative data in the mistaken belief that it is somehow 'easier' to make sense of, write up and publish. However, help is at hand with this slim volume which tackles the subject of data analysis in primary care in a 'user-friendly' way with numerous appropriate worked examples. Each chapter starts with an outline of the specific learning objectives for that chapter against which you can measure your progress, and ends with the answers to the exercises and suggestions for further reading.

In the first chapter Kim Cornish provides a basic introduction to using statistics in research, beginning with some fundamental concepts of statistics such as how to select participants for a particular research project and how one decides whether the data you have collected supports the research hypothesis. Sections on describing and summarising data and how one can measure uncertainty (probability) follow. Choosing the right statistical test is a crucial stage in the analysis of data and Kim gives an excellent overview and practical guide to the different tests available.

In the second chapter Nick Fox and colleagues consider in some detail sampling, not only for quantitative data but also for qualitative data. Again there are numerous worked examples against which you can measure your progress as you work your way through the chapter. To non-statisticians the subject of statistical power often seems a 'black art' whereby sample sizes are somehow arrived at by fearsomely complicated equations. However, in this chapter the topic is dealt with in a clear and practical way. The chapter finishes with a brief review of the statistical power of much general practice research.

The final two chapters by Michael Hewitt consist of a practical step-by-step guide to two of the most commonly used software packages for statistical analysis – Epi Info and SPSS. Data are provided for input into the programme as well as screen shots of expected outputs at each stage. A clear explanation of what the results mean is also given in each section and the chapters are divided into:

- summarising and presenting data

- testing hypotheses
- examining relationships.

By the time you have read these four chapters and worked through the different examples, you should feel more confident about collecting and analysing quantitative data to answer your particular research questions. This should encourage you to become more involved in the primary care research agenda.

CHAPTER ONE

An introduction to using statistics

Kim Cornish

Introduction

Whatever type of research we undertake (for example, naturalistic observation, case study, surveys, or experiments) our efforts can usually generate a considerable amount of data: numbers that represent our research findings and provide the basis for our conclusions. Statistical analyses are the methods most often used to summarise and interpret data. Very often it is the fear of using statistics that prevents us from fully realising the potential of our data. In reality, statistics can be a straightforward and enjoyable process! Knowledge of complex mathematical theories and formulae are not a prerequisite, just confidence in the data and in your own ability to analyse and interpret it.

This chapter is set out to achieve a single aim; to guide you, the researcher, to select the most appropriate statistical test for your data in order to evaluate its significance to your research aims and hypotheses. It is not meant to be an 'all-inclusive' guide to statistical testing but rather a starting point for those who are newcomers to statistical analysis. No mathematical background nor familiarity with research methodology and design are assumed (see Chapter 2 in *Research Approaches in Primary Care*). However, as you become more experienced and confident in the use of statistics you may want to use it as a manual to be 'dipped into' at the appropriate place for your current research project. It should also be noted that although the orientation of this pack will be on 'quantitative data', other types of data (for example, qualitative) are extensively used in research.

Selecting your participants: populations and samples

How you select the participants (alternatively you can use the term 'subjects') for your study is crucial. It can make the difference between a well-designed experimental study, which lends itself to appropriate statistical analysis, and a poorly designed study which, among other things, can affect the statistical analysis used and ultimately the generalisability of the results. It is therefore important that the participants in your study are the most appropriate for your research question. As a researcher you must ensure that, as a group, your participants are not atypical or unrepresentative of the population to which you want to generalise. This advice applies to all types of participant groups, whether they are patients, clients, chiropodists, speech therapists, or some similar group. In order to achieve this you need to consider the distinction between a population and a sample.

Populations and samples

One of the main aims of scientific research is to generalise from examples. As a general practitioner, you might be interested in evaluating the effectiveness of a new therapy or treatment for patients with mental-health problems, while as a health visitor you might want to assess the specific health needs of your caseload. In both cases, the population you want to study should consist of all existing members of that group. In reality, the practical constraints that such a study imposes (for example, finance, time, availability of participants, etc.) usually make it an impossible task. In this context, studying a sample, that is, a subset of the population you are interested in, is a more attainable goal. This allows you to generalise your findings to a particular population. However, in order to achieve this effectively you must ensure that your sample is free from what is referred to as 'sampling bias'. Sampling bias occurs when a sample is unrepresentative of the population to which you want to generalise. This can occur for a number of reasons: first, the range of the sample population is too narrow given the hypothesis under test; second, there is over-representation of one particular category at the expense of other categories; and third, if the sample size is too small then random variation may create a biased sample.

Random samples

To ensure that you are able to generalise from sample to population, one method is to use a simple random sample. By definition, this is a sample in which every member of the target population has an equal chance of being picked and each independent of each other. It is crucial that we ensure that no members of the population have a greater chance than others of getting into our sample. Different types of samples, including random samples, are further described in Chapter 2, Sampling.

Sample size

It is much easier to produce a biased sample with small sample sizes, although in some types of clinical research the subject area dictates the use of small numbers. In the field of clinical neuropsychology, for example, you may be interested in evaluating specific everyday memory deficits in patients with acquired temporal lobe deficits. The rarity of this condition may make it possible for you to gain access to only one or two patients. As a general rule, however, you should aim for the largest sample size possible for your type of data. This issue becomes especially relevant when using a research design that involves collecting data from such methods as questionnaires (structured and semi-structured) and surveys, which if not produced in large enough quantities are more likely to produce a biased response based upon an unrepresentative, small sample size. It is also important to remember that the larger the data set the greater the reliability of the statistical analysis. Importantly, statistical analysis will help you reduce your chance of obtaining random errors in two main ways: first, by ensuring accurate and consistent description of a sample from a target population; and second, by providing a consistent basis for the inference of characteristics of your target population, based on the characteristics of only a sample.

In summary, it is important that from the very onset of your research study you carefully address the issues of composition and size of your sample. As a researcher you must avoid working with samples that are not representative of your target population. You should also ensure that your sample sizes are sufficient to allow appropriate statistical analyses of your data. Following these procedures will increase the likelihood of the ability to draw valid conclusions from your research design and analysis and reduce the risk of misinterpretation due to biased sampling and chance error.

Exercise 1

Poor quality data often derives from asking questions in the wrong way or to the wrong persons. Explain why the following may lead to useless data.

1. In order to investigate the relationship between alcohol consumption and physical fitness in men aged 35 years and over, a sample of 10 males were selected from a local fitness centre in a busy city centre.
2. To determine the relationship between clinical mood states in mental-health patients and the impact of different types of music, the researcher used individuals drawn from an undergraduate student population.

The research hypothesis: how do you decide when the data support it?

At the very core of research is the need to test hypotheses, ideas you may have about how one event might cause another to occur or why events or situations happen the way they do. In scientific research a hypothesis must be clearly stated; it must be testable. It is never enough to justify assertions that have relied solely on common sense or hearsay evidence. Instead, the researcher must test the validity of these assertions by formulating them into testable hypotheses and then, by using appropriate research methodology and statistical analysis, decide whether the results support or refute the research hypothesis.

The first thing you notice about a hypothesis is that it predicts a relationship between two or more events, for instance individuals aged over 70 years will present with an increased number of health problems compared to individuals below the age of 70 years. These events are more typically known as variables. By definition, a variable is anything that varies! In our example, age obviously varies over a wide range of values, from below 70 years to above 70 years. The incidence of health problems is also a variable because individuals can present with varying numbers of problems or none at all. The list of potential variables in any study is endless (height, weight, age at testing, time to respond to a situation or test, fitness level, blood pressure count, response to medication, level of anxiety, depression etc.). However, what is crucial to remember is that in order to carry out a test of your hypothesis, it must in principle be possible for your predicted relationship to occur or not occur. So, while in our example we predict that there will be a relationship between age and incidence of health problems, we must also accept the possibility that there will be no relationship between age and incidence of health problems. This statement of no difference or relationship between the two variables is known as the 'null hypothesis', which predicts that any difference, or relationship, found between two sets of results are due to chance fluctuations in participants' behaviour rather than to any 'real' difference or relationship between the two variables.

It is the role of statistical analysis to demonstrate that a difference is large enough to support the research hypothesis. Statistical analyses indicate the probability that you can reject the null hypothesis and accept the research hypothesis that there is a 'real' difference or relationship between your two variables. As previously noted, the question you are typically asking when you use statistical analyses is whether or not the results you obtained from your sample can be generalised to your target population. So, in our example, if you observed a relationship between increased age and increased incidence of health problems, the null hypothesis would state that the relationship had occurred as a result of chance variation in your sample data and could therefore not be generalised to a population of all men and women over the age of 70 years. In contrast, the research hypothesis would state that the relationship is statistically meaningful, and can therefore be generalised to the target population.

What is also important to consider, however, is that having to accept the null hypothesis rather than reject it does not mean your research has *failed*. Retaining the null hypothesis can often tell you important information about how your participants performed, or it can help you critically assess the design of your research study and help you look for weaknesses within it (for example, small sample size, poor research design, inappropriate statistical test etc.).

Exercise 2

Identify the research hypothesis and null hypothesis from the following examples.

1. There will be a difference in levels of stress and burnout experienced among three different primary healthcare professionals: GPs, health visitors and speech therapists.
2. That there will be no difference in levels of stress and burnout among the different primary healthcare professionals.
3. In a sample of patients characterised by their familial predisposition to high blood pressure, it was hypothesised that the number of capillaries per unit volume of tissue would be reduced compared with a similar sample of patients with no familial predisposition to high blood pressure.
4. There would be no difference in the reduction in number of capillaries per unit volume of tissue between patients with a familial predisposition to high blood pressure and those with no familial predisposition to high blood pressure.

Describing and summarising data

By the time you start this stage, you have selected your participant sample, identified your research hypothesis, and used the appropriate experimental design to test the research hypothesis (*see* Chapter 2 in *Research Approaches in Primary Care*). You now have, in your possession, some actual raw data! By data, we refer to the reduction of the actual results of a study into numerical format. This is the first, preliminary step in the statistical analysis of your data. However, what is particularly crucial at this stage is that you address the issue of what type of data you have.

Levels of measurement

Traditionally, data are assigned to one of four hierarchical measurement categories. The levels of measurement from lower to higher are nominal, ordinal, interval and ratio.

Nominal-scale (categorical) measurement is used when the items to be measured can be organised into exclusive and exhaustive categories that cannot be compared numerically. Gender and marital status are examples of nominal data. An individual may be married or not married, but cannot be more married than another. You may, for example, want to classify mental-health patients in terms of their diagnoses, giving the label 'manic-depressive' to one patient and 'paranoid schizophrenic' to another and so on. This type of data is solely descriptive: a patient either has or does not have any particular diagnosis.

The next level of measurement uses the *ordinal scale*. This scale is used when the data to be measured can be ranked or ordered. Many questionnaires seek data at this level of measurement. For example, a satisfaction questionnaire might have response categories of 'excellent', 'good', 'average', 'poor' and 'very poor'. A person who judges a service to be 'good' is clearly more satisfied than one who responds 'poor'. The data for this measurement scale can be ranked, although it is not possible to state that the differences between successive scale categories are exactly equal. Thus, the difference in satisfaction between an individual who responds 'poor' and one who responds 'average' may not be the same as the difference in satisfaction between a person who responds 'good' and one who responds 'excellent'.

Interval scales refer to data where distances between intervals of measurement are equal and the data are part of a continuum of values. An example of an interval scale is temperature as measured by Fahrenheit or centigrade. It is possible to say that the temperature difference between 10°C and 20°C is the same as the difference between 110°C and 120°C. Interval scales are similar to the highest level of measurement, ratio scales, except they do not have a true zero point. The lowest point on the centigrade scale is not 0°C since lower temperatures are measurable. Consequently, it is *not* true to say that something at 20°C is twice as hot as a similar item at 10°C.

Ratio scales have all the attributes of interval scales but also have absolute zero points. A person's height, weight and age are all examples of ratio-level data. This form of data enables ratio comparisons to be performed: it *is* possible to say that one person is twice as heavy as another, one-and-a-half times taller, or three times as old.

Higher levels of measurement enable more sophisticated statistical analyses. It is always advisable to collect your data in such a way as to maintain the highest possible level. When collecting peoples' weights, for example, using the categories of 'above average', 'average' and 'below average' (ordinal scale measurement) will allow less sophisticated statistical analyses than using the actual values in kilograms (ratio scale measurement). The data can always be collapsed into useful categories at a later date if necessary.

Organising your data: descriptive statistics

Quantitative data

Once you have described the data provided by your participants by assigning numbers to them, the next step is to reduce this larger mass of information to a smaller and more manageable base of information. To do this, researchers typically use what are referred to as 'measures of central tendency', which allow you to summarise data by a single, central score. Whenever we collect data there is always a high probability that most scores or responses will fall in the centre of a distribution and that relatively few scores will fall at the extremes. The distribution in the population of height, weight and blood pressure demonstrates this point well. Three measures of central tendency are typically used to express this central point of distribution: 'mean', 'median' and 'mode'.

You may well be familiar with the first of these concepts, the mean, which refers to an arithmetic average. Each score from the distribution is added and then the sum is divided by the total number of scores. To illustrate this, say we wanted to know the mean score on a measure that assessed risk of self-injurious behaviour in a sample of 10 young mothers suffering from a post-natal illness. Their individual risk scores are as follows:

69   60   55   72   62   53   63   63   58   57

If n stands for the number of scores, Σ (Greek capital letter 'sigma') stands for 'the sum of', and x stands for raw scores, then:

$$mean = \frac{\Sigma x}{n}$$

$$mean = \frac{69 + 60 + 55 + 72 + 62 + 53 + 63 + 63 + 58 + 57}{10}$$

$$mean = 61.2$$

The principle advantage of knowing the mean is that it acts as a prerequisite for other, more complex statistical analyses. The mean is also one of the few statistical operations understood by the general public. However, its main disadvantage is that it can be too sensitive towards extreme scores. So, for example, if you had rated on a scale of 1–7 eight mothers-to-be's attitude towards home delivery of their baby versus a hospital delivery, and their scores were 1 1 1 1 1 1 7 9, the mean of 2.75 would reflect a number that is higher than the rating of six of the eight people surveyed. Clearly extreme scores can distort the mean and this becomes more prominent when the size of distribution is small, as in our example.

The median, in contrast to the mean, is less sensitive to extreme scores and represents the point that divides the distribution of scores into two equal halves. In order to do this, however, the scores must first be arranged in increasing order. To find the median in our previous example we first list the scores:

53   55   57   58   60   62   63   63   69   72

When the number of observations in the distribution is odd, the median is easy to calculate, you just take the middle score. However, since there are 10 scores in total here, our median lies between the fifth and sixth scores (60 and 62 respectively). To calculate the median, we add 60 and 62 together and divide by 2. The median in this example is therefore 61. A main disadvantage of the median, however, is that it does not use all the information in the data and can be difficult to calculate.

The third measure, the mode, is perhaps the least reliable of all three central tendency measures. The mode represents the most frequently occurring score in a distribution and is useful for categorical data. In our example, the mode is 63. More participants had a weight of 63 kilograms than any other weight measure. Fortunately, the majority of distributions are unimodal, that is, one score occurs more frequently than others. Less often, there is a bimodal distribution when a number of scores appear more than once. The main disadvantage of this measure is that it takes into account the least information about the distribution of scores.

Table 1.1   Table for calculation of odds ratios

	Diseased (case)	No disease (control)
Exposed	a	b
Not exposed	c	d

Table 1.2   Data showing association between exposure and outcome in a case-control study of the effects of smoking on lung disease

	Died of lung cancer	Did not die of lung cancer
Smokers	36	21 353
Non-smokers	1	3093

Categorical data

When you do not have a continuous variable as an outcome and instead have discrete data, i.e. binary/dichotomous variables as outcomes and predictors, you may still want a summary measure of association. For this, you can use an odds ratio (OR).

If a, b, c and d are the number of individuals in each cell (not in proportions) then the odds ratio is (a×b)/(b×c).

So, for example, if you wanted to describe an association between exposure and outcome in a case-control study of the effects of smoking on lung cancer, you could place the data into a two-by-two table as shown in Table 1.2.

Calculation of the odds ratio would be ((36×3093)/(1×21 353)) = 5.21, indicating that the odds of dying from lung cancer are more than five times greater for those who smoke than for those who don't.

Measures of variability

When we reduce a large set of numbers to an average score (see mean, median and mode) we discard a lot of very useful and potentially important information. Suppose, for example, you want to assess the relationship between weight gain and eating patterns in a sample of 10 adults with a family history of cardiac problems. The mean weight (kilograms) was calculated as 61.2, although you notice that individual weight measures ranged from 53–72 kilograms. This variability in scores around the mean clearly demonstrates that measures of central tendency do not tell us everything we need to know about an individual's score. We also need a measure of the variability of scores around that mean. As we shall see, calculating how much each individual score deviates from the mean can do this.

The most commonly used procedures for calculating the variability in data are the standard deviation and variance. These take into account every score in the distribution and are relatively simple to calculate. The first step is to calculate deviation scores (d). This is achieved by subtracting the mean from each raw score in the distribution. This will leave you with a set of deviations, some of which may be negative. However, as the sum of these deviations will always be zero, the second step of the analysis involves squaring each deviation (d²). These are then added up and the sum is divided by the number of deviation scores minus one (n–1). The square root (√) is then obtained:

$$SD = \sqrt{\frac{\Sigma d^2}{n-1}}$$

In our example of weight distribution, the deviation scores and squared deviation scores are shown in Table 1.3.

The standard deviation (SD) would be calculated as follows:

$$SD = \sqrt{\frac{\Sigma d^2}{n-1}}$$

(i) Σd^2 = 67.24 + 38.44 + 17.64 + 10.24 + 1.44 + 0.64 + 3.24 + 3.24 + 60.84 + 116.64 = 319.6

(ii) $\frac{319.6}{9}$ = 35.51   (this represents the variance)

(iii) SD   = $\sqrt{35.51}$ = 5.96 kg

Table 1.3   Computation of the deviation scores and the squared deviation scores for sets of weight scores in adults with a family history of cardiac problems

Weight (kilograms)	Mean score	Deviation score (d)	Squared deviation score (d²)
53	61.2	–8.2	67.24
55	61.2	–6.2	38.44
57	61.2	–4.2	17.64
58	61.2	–3.2	10.24
60	61.2	–1.2	1.44
62	61.2	0.8	0.64
63	61.2	1.8	3.24
63	61.2	1.8	3.24
69	61.2	7.8	60.84
72	61.2	10.8	116.64
			Σd^2 = 319.6

Thus, the mean weight of our sample is 61.2 kilograms with a SD around the mean of 5.96 kilograms. As a general rule, the larger the standard deviation, the more spread the scores in the distribution, and the smaller the standard deviation, the more central the scores in the distribution.

Normal distribution

The normal distribution represents one of the most useful tools in statistics. If plotted on a graph such as a histogram, the distribution of your data should resemble a bell-shaped curve, rounded at the top and tapering off at each end. The majority of scores should always fall towards the centre of the distribution, which represents the mean, median and mode; the farther a score is away from the mean, the less likely it is to occur. However, not all distributions are normal, in that they can be skewed, or lopsided either to the left or the right of the mode (most frequent value) of the distribution. One of the most frequent reasons for this occurring in experimental research is because of either 'floor effects' or 'ceiling effects'. A 'floor effect' will positively skew the distribution (to the left) and this typically appears when the majority of participants have failed or misinterpreted answers or responses to questions or tests. In contrast, a 'ceiling effect' which negatively skews the distribution (to the right) appears when the majority of participants find the questions, test items etc. too easy, thus placing an artificial ceiling or limit on how well they do. If you are unsure about the distribution of scores in your own data, plot a normal distribution. As you will see later, the more powerful statistics (known as 'parametric statistics') require, as a prerequisite, that your data be normally distributed.

Table 1.4 gives an example of a set of data that, when plotted, approximates to a normal distribution. The data are for length of consultations between a GP and her patients. The original data for time taken for consultations have been grouped into a frequency table so that rows one and two show that no consultations took less than two minutes, row three shows that one consultation took between two and three minutes, and so on.

The plotted histogram of this data is shown in Figure 1.1, with a normal distribution curve overlaid.

The data show that from 219 consultations, Dr Green spent an average of approximately 10.3 minutes with each patient and that typically, a consultation took between 9 and 9.9 minutes (mode).

Exercise 3

Find the means and SDs of the male participants' score and the female participants' score in Table 1.5. Is there a difference in means and standard deviations across the two groups?

Table 1.4   Length (in minutes) of patient consultations for Dr Green

Consultation time (minutes)	Number of patients (frequency)
0–0.9	0
1–1.9	0
2–2.9	1
3–3.9	1
4–4.9	1
5–5.9	8
6–6.9	16
7–7.9	25
8–8.9	29
9–9.9	30
10–10.9	26
11–11.9	22
12–12.9	18
13–13.9	14
14–14.9	10
15–15.9	8
16–16.9	5
17–17.9	3
18–18.9	1
19–19.9	1

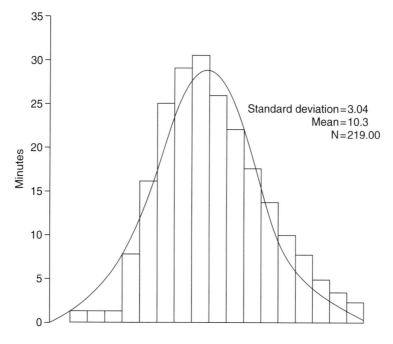

Figure 1.1   Histogram showing frequency of length of patient consultations for Dr Green.

Table 1.5   **Daily intake of fat grams in a sample of young males and females**

Male participants	Daily fat intake (grams)	Female participants	Daily fat intake (grams)
1	80	6	51
2	72	7	65
3	95	8	53
4	79	9	75
5	69	10	40
mean		mean	
SD		SD	

Probability: a measure of uncertainty

Understanding the concept of probability is crucial to understanding statistics in research. A statistical test is simply a means of calculating the probability that your results are due to chance fluctuations. If this chance probability is very low, then you can reject the null hypothesis that the differences are chance differences. Instead you can accept the research hypothesis that your results are statistically significant and not likely to have occurred as a result of chance fluctuations. It is crucial, however, that you do not place too much importance on the term 'statistically significant', which should never be confused with the term 'clinically significant'. For example, improvement in the attention capacity of a group of attention deficit hyperactivity disorder (ADHD) children from 30 seconds to 90 seconds using a new behavioural technique would only be of clinical significance if the results could be improved over a much wider time range, say from 30 seconds to 5 minutes. The initial change from 30 seconds to 90 seconds may well be statistically significant, but this finding may not be of any great importance in a clinical sense.

Selecting a level of significance

You need to decide what risk you are prepared to take that the scores resulting from your study occurred by chance. It is impossible to be 100% certain. So are you prepared to accept a 99% probability that your results represent a real difference against a 1% probability that they occurred by chance? If you are, then you adopt a significance level of 0.01 (a 1 in 100 chance) which means that the difference in your results will be assumed to reflect chance fluctuations unless the results could only arise by chance once in 100 or less. However, you may be prepared to accept a 95% probability that your results represent a real difference against a 5% probability that they occurred by chance. If you are, then you adopt a significance level of 0.05 (a 1 in 20 chance), which is traditionally the highest level of probability to accept as statistically significant.

It is up to you to decide which level of significance you wish to apply to your results (0.01 or 0.05). For this reason, the researcher must always state the significance level used to accept or reject the null hypothesis. The way this is expressed is to state that the probability of the result being due to chance is less than 1% ($p<0.01$) or less than 5% ($p<0.05$). This is why you often see in academic or clinical journals the statement 'the results of the study indicated a significant difference ($p<0.05$) between the groups (or conditions)'. Sometimes you also see other probability levels quoted, such as $p<0.001$ or $p<0.02$. These indicate probabilities of 1 in a 1000 (0.001) or 2 in a 100 (0.02) of your results occurring by chance.

To summarise, the null hypothesis is only rejected if the probability of your results or ones more extreme is less than or equal to ($\leq$) the significance level 0.05. If the probability of your results is greater than ($>$) 0.05 (i.e. 0.06, 0.08, 0.10, 0.12, 0.20 etc.) then you fail to reject the null hypothesis. This is known as a 'non-significant result' and indicates that any differences in your data reflect chance fluctuations rather than real statistical differences. However, in order to determine whether your result is significant or non-significant, you must first calculate the appropriate 'statistic' for the statistical test you are applying. This will be addressed in the next section.

Exercise 4

Suppose that a researcher reports that a significant difference ($p<0.01$) has been found between the effectiveness of two types of incontinence pads.

1. Which of the following are correct?
    The null hypothesis can be rejected because the probability of the difference being due to chance is less than 1 in 100 (1%), 1 in 20 (5%) and 1 in 1000 (0.1%).
2. Which of the above would indicate the greatest level of significance?

Dealing with data: how to choose the right statistical test

After the initial step of organising your data has been accomplished, you are now ready to analyse the data in order to test for statistical significance.

Be aware that at first glance the sheer number of tests can seem staggering and confusing. However, it is the goal of the researcher to select the one most appropriate to the design of the study and the type of data collected. The statistic derived from this test will then enable you to determine the probability of your results occurring by chance.

Statistical tests fall into two main categories: non-parametric tests and parametric tests. It is crucial that you fully appreciate the difference between these categories of statistical tests because the type of data required for each varies. Non-parametric tests require data to be either at ordinal level (only capable of being ranked in order of magnitude) or at nominal level (categorical data). In contrast, parametric tests require data to be of at least interval level. The tests that comprise this category are often said to be more 'powerful' because they can take more information into account about the difference between scores. Consequently, these tests require that your sample data be drawn from a normally distributed population and that there is homogeneity of variance, that is, that variances of the samples are not significantly different. These latter two assumptions are not required for non-parametric analysis.

It is also important that you consider the experimental design of your study (see Chapter 2 in *Research Approaches in Primary Care*) before deciding on the statistical test. Certain tasks can only incorporate data that fall within a related design (also known as 'within-subjects' or 'repeated measures design'), whilst others only incorporate data that fall within an unrelated design (also known as 'between-subjects' or 'independent measures design').

The use of computers in statistical analysis

With today's computer technology there is virtually no need to perform statistical analyses by hand. Although all the tests described in this section can be performed manually, the dramatic rise in the availability of computer statistical packages over the past 15 years (for example, SPSS-PC; SPSS for Windows; MINITAB etc.) has meant that the majority of statistical analysis can now be performed by computer. It is often much simpler to let a computer program do the work and many of the current packages have the added bonus of being easy to use, versatile and widely available. For this reason, it is assumed in this section that you have access to a computer package that will allow you to store, process and analyse data. (Warning: be aware that computers will analyse anything! It is up to the researcher to check that data and results are sensible.) For this reason, the reader, whether a novice or more experienced researcher, is strongly recommended to refer to Chapter 3 *An introduction to using SPSS* and Chapter 4 *An introduction to using Epi Info*.

When to use the tests

Non-parametric tests

Chi-squared Test
Use when data are nominal (categorical) and all data are counts. Because data from the same individual cannot be allocated to more than one category, this test can only be used in an unrelated design. The statistic is written as χ^2.

Rationale: To determine whether two proportions could have occurred by chance.

Example: Prevalence of cough in 110 adult males, of whom 55 are smokers and 55 non-smokers.

Mann-Whitney U Test

Use when data are ordinal (rank ordered) and the design is unrelated. The statistic is written as U.

Rationale: To determine differences in medians could have occurred by chance.

Example: Fifteen adults with a persistent back complaint were offered one of two treatments: aromatherapy or medication. Seven chose aromatherapy and eight chose medication. Two weeks later they were asked to rate the perceived beneficial effects of their chosen treatment.

Wilcoxon Signed Rank Test

Use when data are ordinal (rank ordered) and the design is related. The statistic is written as W.

Rationale: To determine whether differences in scores of one group or matched differences could have occurred by chance.

Example: A group of adults with a persistent back complaint were each given two treatments: aromatherapy and medication. Half of the group received aromatherapy first and half medication first. Two weeks after their first treatment they were asked to rate its beneficial effects on a 10-point scale. They were then given the second treatment and again after two weeks were asked to rate its beneficial effects.

Kruskal-Wallis Test

Often considered as an extension of the Mann-Whitney U Test. Use when data are ordinal and the design is unrelated. The statistic is written as H.

Rationale: To determine whether differences in the scores of three or more groups under one condition could have occurred by chance.

Example: Assessment of vocabulary development in three different age groups of preschool children: 18–24 months, 2–3 years and 3–4 years.

Friedman Test

Use when data are ordinal and the design is related. The statistic is written as Xr^2.

Rationale: To determine whether the differences in scores of one group under three or more conditions could have occurred by chance.

Example: Assessment of three different aspects of language development (standardised measures of comprehension, vocabulary and speech) in a group of 3–4 year-olds.

Spearman's Rho Test

This is a correlational test and should be used when data are ordinal. The numbers used to express correlation are called correlation coefficients. If two measures are in perfect association, i.e. individuals who rate highly on one aspect of behaviour always rate highly on another, and when one aspect of behaviour is absent, then the other also is absent, you have a perfect positive correlation. This is expressed as a coefficient of $+1$. If, on the other hand, there is no association whatsoever between two variables, you have zero correlation and can assign the number 0. In the majority of cases, however, associations fall along intermediate stages between 0 and $+1$. The statistic is written as r_s.

Rationale: To determine the amount and significance of a correlation between two variables.

Example: The relationship between weight gain and levels of exercise on an ordinal scale.

Parametric tests

t-Test for unrelated data
Use when data are at interval level and the parametric assumptions have been met (see above). The statistic is written as t.

Rationale: To determine whether the mean scores of two groups are significantly different. Its non-parametric equivalent is the Mann-Whitney U Test (see above).

t-Test for related data
Use when data are at interval level and the parametric assumptions have been met (see above). The statistic is written as t.

Rationale: To determine whether the mean scores of one group are significantly different under two conditions. Its non-parametric equivalent is the Wilcoxon Signed Rank Test (see above).

Pearson Product Moment Correlation
Use when data are at interval level and the parametric assumptions have been met (see above). The statistic is written as r.

Rationale: To determine the amount and significance of a correlation between two variables. Its non-parametric equivalent is the Spearman's Rho Test (see above).

Analysis of Variance for unrelated data (One-way)
Use when data are at interval level and the parametric assumptions have been met (see above). The statistic is written as F.

Rationale: To determine whether the mean scores of three groups are significantly different. Its non-parametric equivalent is the Kruskal-Wallis Test (see above).

Analysis of Variance for related data (One-way)
Use when data are at interval level and the parametric assumptions have been met (see above). The statistic is written as F.

Rationale: To determine whether the mean scores for one group are significantly different under three conditions. Its non-parametric equivalent is the Friedman Test (see above).

Exercise 5

1. Identify the most appropriate non-parametric statistical test for the following research design.

    Incidence of human papilloma virus infection in young women under the age of 25 years was assessed by two samples of participants: medical students (N = 30) and student nurses (N = 40). Of the medical students 65% identified the four main risk factors compared to 40% of student nurses.

2. Identify the most appropriate parametric statistical test for the following research design.

    The number of recent stressful life events was compared in two samples of patients: 95 patients suffering from cardiovascular disease on a general practice list and a control group of 80 orthopaedic patients from the same list.

Interpreting data

Once you have applied the appropriate statistical test, the 'statistic' (for instance, t from the t-Test, U from the Mann-Whitney U Test etc.) will then be evaluated to see how significant it is. On the basis of this result you either accept or reject the null hypothesis. If the null hypothesis has been rejected, the conclusion is that the research hypothesis can be taken as correct. However, even at this stage, problems can still occur in the interpretation of results. Two types of errors have been identified. One type concerns drawing a conclusion when you should not (*Type I error*), and the second not drawing a conclusion when you should (*Type II error*). Type I and Type II errors are discussed further in Chapter 2, *Sampling*.

As mentioned previously, it is also important to distinguish between statistical significance and *clinical significance*, which refers to whether a result is of any clinical importance. You need to remember that a statistical test can only tell you the probability that any difference in your results did not occur by chance fluctuations. It does not tell you how large the difference is, nor whether the difference is great enough to be of clinical importance. One of our main goals as researchers should be to focus on the practical implications of our work as well as its statistical significance.

Conclusion

The aim of this chapter has been to provide you, the researcher, with an overview of the different types of statistical tests used in quantitative data analysis and their application to research. As stated in the introduction to this chapter, it is not an all-inclusive guide to statistical testing but rather an introduction for you to expand upon as you become more experienced in research design and methodology.

Answers to exercises

Exercise 1

1. Sample size is very small (N = 10) and unrepresentative of the target population (participants selected from only one gym and in geographical location).
2. Sample size is very small (N = 7) and unrepresentative of the target population (participants recruited from an undergraduate population and there is no evidence to indicate any of the actual participants had been diagnosed as having mental-health problems).

Exercise 2

1. Research hypothesis.
2. Null hypothesis.
3. Research hypothesis.
4. Null hypothesis.

Exercise 3

1. Males: mean 79 (SD 9.0).
2. Females: mean 56.8 (SD 12.1).
    The difference lies in a higher male than female mean, although the SD of the female mean suggests a larger distribution of scores compared to the SD of the male mean.

Exercise 4

1. 1 in 100.
2. 1 in 1000.

Exercise 5

1. Chi-Square Test.
2. t-Test (unrelated).

Further reading

Clegg F (1990) *Simple Statistics*. Cambridge University Press, Cambridge.

Clifford C and Harkin L (1997) *Inferential Statistics in Nursing and Healthcare*. OLF/Churchill Livingstone, Edinburgh.

Greene J and D'Olivera M (1982) *Learning to Use Statistical Tests in Psychology*. Oxford University Press, Oxford.

Hicks C M (1990) *Research and Statistics: A Practical Introduction for Nurses*. Prentice Hall, London.

Kinnear P R and Gray C D (1997) *SPSS for Windows Made Simple* (2e). Psychology Press, Hove.

Swinscow T D V (1996) *Statistics at Square One* (9e) (revised by M J Campbell). BMJ Publishing Group, London.

CHAPTER TWO

Sampling

Nick Fox, Amanda Hunn and Nigel Mathers

Introduction

Sampling and sample size are crucial issues in pieces of quantitative research, which seek to make statistically based generalisations from the study results to the wider world. To generalise in this way, it is essential that both the sampling method used and the sample size are appropriate, such that the results are representative, and that the statistics can discern associations or differences within the results of a study.

Having successfully completed this chapter, you will be able to:

- distinguish between random and non-random methods of sample selection
- describe the advantages of random sample selection
- identify the different methods of random sample selection
- match the appropriate methods of sample selection to the research question and design
- describe the factors influencing sample size
- decide upon an appropriate sample size.

Working through this chapter

The study time involved in this chapter is approximately 10 hours. In addition to the written text, the chapter includes exercises. It is suggested that as you work through the chapter, you establish for yourself a 'reflective log', linking the work in the chapter to your own research interests and needs, and documenting your reflections on the ethnographic method. Include your responses to the exercises plus your own thoughts as you read and consider the material.

The representative sample

It is an explicit or implicit objective of most studies in healthcare which 'count' something or other (quantitative studies) to offer conclusions that are generalisable. This means that the findings of a study apply to situations other than that of the cases in the study. To give a hypothetical example, Smith and Jones' (1997) study of consultation rates in primary care, based on data from five practices in differing geographic settings (urban, suburban, rural), finds higher rates in the urban environment. When they wrote it up for publication, Smith and Jones used statistics to claim their findings could be generalised: the differences applied not just to these five practices, but to all practices in the country.

For such a claim to be legitimate (technically, for the study to possess 'external validity'), the authors must persuade us that their sample was not biased: that it was representative. Although other criteria must also be met (for instance, that the design was both appropriate and carried out correctly – the study's 'internal validity' and 'reliability'), it is the representativeness of a sample which allows the researcher to generalise the findings to the wider population. (If a study has an unrepresentative or biased sample, then it may still have internal validity and reliability, but it will not possess external validity. Consequently the results of the study will be applicable only to the group under study.)

So it is essential to a study's design (assuming that study wants to generalise and is not simply descriptive of one setting) that sampling is taken seriously. The first part of this chapter looks at how to gather a 'representative' sample which gives a study external validity and permits valid generalisation.

However, there is a second issue which must be addressed in relation to sampling, and this is predominantly a question of sample size. Generalisations from data to wider population depend upon a kind of statistic which tests inferences or hypotheses. For instance, an inferential statistic known as the 't-Test' is used to test a hypothesis that there is a difference between two populations, based on a sample from each. To give an example, we select 100 males and 100 females and test their body mass index. We find a difference in our samples, and wish to argue that that difference is not an accident but reflects an actual difference in the wider populations from which the samples were drawn. We use a t-Test to see if we can make this claim legitimately.

Most people know that the larger a sample size, the more likely it is that finding a difference such as this is not due to chance, but really does mean there is a difference between men and women. Unfortunately, recent research (Fox and Mathers 1997) has shown that many quantitative studies undertaken and published in medical journals do not have a sufficient sample size to adequately test the hypothesis which the study was designed to explore. Such studies are of little use, and – for example in the case of drug trials – could be dangerous if their findings were generalised.

We will consider these issues of sample size, and how to calculate an adequate size for a study sample, in the second half of this chapter. Before that, let us think in greater detail about what a sample is.

Why do we need to select a sample anyway?

In some circumstances it is not necessary to select a sample. If the subjects of your study are very rare, for instance a disease occurring only once in 100 000 children, then you might decide to study every case you can find. More usually, however, you are likely to find yourself in a situation where the potential subjects of your study are much more common and you cannot practically include everybody. For example, a study of everybody in the UK who had been diagnosed as suffering from asthma would be impossible: it would take too long and cost too much money.

So it is necessary to find some way of reducing the number of subjects included in the study without biasing the findings in any way. Random sampling is one way of achieving this, and with appropriate statistics such a study can yield generalisable findings at far lower cost. Samples can also be taken using non-random techniques, but in this chapter we will emphasise random sampling, which – if conducted adequately – will ensure external validity.

Random sampling

To obtain a random (or probability) sample, the first step is to define the population from which it is to be drawn. This population is known as the *sampling frame.* For instance, you are interested in doing a study of children aged between two and 10 years diagnosed within the last month as having otitis media. Or you want to study adults (aged 16–65 years) diagnosed as having asthma and receiving drug treatment for asthma in the last six months, and living in a defined geographical region. In each case, these limits define the sampling frame. If the research design is based on an experimental design, such as a randomised controlled trial (RCT), with two or more groups, then the population frame may often be very tightly defined with strict eligibility criteria.

Within an RCT, potential subjects are randomly allocated to either the intervention (treatment) group or the control group. By randomly allocating subjects to each of the groups, potential differences between the comparison groups will be negated. In this way confounding variables (i.e. variables you haven't thought of, or controlled for) will be equally distributed between each of the groups and will be less likely to influence the outcome or dependent variables in either of the groups.

Randomisation within an experimental design is a way of ensuring control over confounding variables and as such it allows the researcher to have a greater confidence in identifying real associations between an independent variable (the cause) and a dependent variable (the effect or outcome measure).

The term *random* may imply to you that it is possible to take some sort of haphazard or *ad hoc* approach, for example stopping the first 20 people you meet in the street for inclusion in your study. This is not random in the true sense of the word. To be a random sample, every individual in the population must have an equal probability of being selected. In order to carry out random sampling properly, strict procedures need to be adhered to.

Random sampling techniques can be split into *simple random sampling* and *systematic random sampling.*

Simple random sampling

If selections are made purely by chance, this is known as simple random sampling. So, for instance, if we had a population containing 5000 people, we could allocate every individual a different number. If we wanted to achieve a sample size of 200, we could achieve this by pulling 200 of the 5000 numbers out of a hat. Another way of selecting the numbers would be to use a table of random numbers. These tables are usually to be found in the appendices of most statistical textbooks.

Simple random sampling, although technically valid, is a very laborious way of carrying out sampling. A simpler and quicker way is to use systematic random sampling.

Systematic random sampling

Systematic random sampling is a more commonly employed method. After numbers are allocated to everybody in the population frame, the first individual is picked using a random number table and then subsequent subjects are selected using a fixed sampling interval, i.e. every nth person.

Assume, for example, that we wanted to carry out a survey of patients with asthma attending clinics in one city. There may be too many to interview everyone, so we want to select a representative sample. If there are 3000 people attending the clinics in total and we only require a sample of 200, we would need to:

- calculate the sampling interval by dividing 3000 by 200 to give a sampling fraction of 15
- select a random number between one and 15 using a set of random tables
- if this number were 13, we select the individual allocated number 13 and then go on to select every 15th person.

This will give us a total sample size of 200 as required.

Care needs to be taken when using a systematic random sampling method in case there is some bias in the way that lists of individuals are compiled. For example, if all the husbands' names precede wives' names and the sampling interval is an even number, then we may end up selecting all women and no men.

Stratified random sampling

Stratified random sampling is a way of ensuring that particular strata or categories of individuals are represented in the sampling process.

If, for example, we want to study consultation rates in a general practice, and we know that approximately 4% of our population frame is made up of a particular ethnic minority group, there is a chance that with simple or systematic random sampling we could end up with no ethnic minorities (or a much-reduced proportion) in our sample. If we wanted to ensure that our sample was representative of the population frame, then we would employ a stratified sampling method.

1. First we would split the population into the different strata, in this case, separating out those individuals with the relevant ethnic background.
2. We would then apply random sampling techniques to each of the two ethnic groups separately, using the same sampling interval in each group.
3. This would ensure that the final sampling frame was representative of the minority group we wanted to include, on a pro rata basis with the actual population.

Disproportionate sampling

Taking this example once more, if our objective was to compare the results of our minority group with the larger group, then we would have difficulty in doing so, using the proportionate stratified sampling just described. This is because the numbers achieved in the minority group, although pro rata those of the population, would not be large enough to demonstrate statistical differences.

To compare the survey results of the minority individuals with those of the larger group, it is necessary to use a disproportionate sampling method. With disproportionate sampling, the strata are not selected pro rata to their size in the wider population. For instance, if we are interested in comparing the referral rates for particular minority groups with other larger groups, then it is necessary to over-sample the smaller categories in order to achieve statistical power, that is, in order to be able to demonstrate statistically significant differences between groups.

Note that, if subsequently we wish to refer to the total sample as a whole; representative of the wider population, then it will become necessary to re-weight the categories back into the proportions in which they are represented in reality. For example, if we wanted to compare the views and satisfaction levels of women who gave birth at home compared with the majority of women who gave birth in hospital, a systematic random sample, although representative of all women giving birth, would not produce a sufficient number of women giving birth at home to be able to compare the results, unless the total sample was so big that it would take many years to collate. We would also end up interviewing more women than we needed who have given birth in hospital. In this case it would be necessary to over-sample or over-represent those women giving birth at home to have enough individuals in each group in order to compare them. We would therefore use disproportionate stratified random sampling to select the sample.

The important thing to note here about disproportionate sampling is that randomisation is still taking place within each stratum or category. So we would use systematic random selection to select a sample from the majority group and the same process to select samples from the minority groups.

Cluster sampling

Cluster sampling is a method frequently employed in national surveys where it is uneconomic to carry out interviews with individuals scattered across the country. Cluster sampling allows individuals to be selected in geographical batches. So, for instance, before selecting at random, the researcher may decide to focus on certain towns, electoral wards or general practices. Multi-stage sampling allows the individuals within the selected cluster units to then be selected at random.

Obviously care must be taken to ensure that the cluster units selected are generally representative of the population and are not strongly biased in any way. If, for example, all the general practices selected for a study were fundholding, this would not be representative of all general practice.

Non-random sampling

Non-random (or non-probability) sampling is not used very often in quantitative social research, but it is increasingly used in market research and commissioned studies. The technique most commonly used is known as quota sampling.

Quota sampling

Quota sampling is a technique whereby the researcher decides in advance on certain key characteristics which s/he will use to stratify the sample. Interviewers are often set sample quotas in terms of age and sex. So, for example, with a sample of 200 people, they may decide that 50% should be male and 50% should be female; and 40% should be aged over 40 years and 60% aged 39 years or less. The difference with a stratified sample is that the respondents in a quota sample are not randomly selected within the strata. The respondents may be selected just because they are accessible to the interviewer. Because random sampling is not employed, it is not possible to apply inferential statistics and generalise the findings to a wider population.

Convenience or opportunistic sampling

Selecting respondents purely because they are easily accessible is known as convenience sampling. Whilst this technique is generally frowned upon by quantitative researchers, it is regarded as an acceptable approach when using a qualitative design, since general-isability is not a main aim of qualitative approaches.

Exercise 1

Read the descriptions below and decide what type of sample selection has taken place.

1. Schoolchildren, some with asthma and some without, are identified from GP records. Method: children are selected randomly within each of the two groups and the number of children in each group is representative of the total patient population for this age group.
2. Children with and without chronic asthma are identified from GP records. Method: the children are selected so that exactly 50% have chronic asthma and 50% have no asthma. Within each group, the children are randomly selected.
3. A survey of the attitudes of mothers with children under one year. Method: inter-viewers stop likely-looking women pushing prams in the street. The number of respondents who fall into different age bands and social classes is strictly controlled.
4. A survey of attitudes of drug users to rehabilitation services. Method: drug users are recruited by advertising in the local newspaper for potential respondents.
5. A postal survey of the attitudes of males to use of male contraceptives. Method: all male adults whose national insurance numbers end in '5' are selected for a survey.
6. A study of the length of stay of patients at Anytown General Hospital. Method: all patients admitted to wards 3, 5, and 10 in a hospital are selected for a study.

Sampling in qualitative research

Since the objective of qualitative research is to understand and give meaning to a social process, rather than quantify and generalise to a wider population, it is inappropriate to use random sampling or apply statistical tests. Sample sizes used in qualitative research are usually very small and the application of statistical tests would be neither appropriate nor feasible.

Qualitative data are often collected using a convenience or opportunistic sampling approach, for instance where the researcher selects volunteers amongst his or her work colleagues. This is rather a haphazard method with potential biases, and many qualitative researchers employ a 'purposive' sample to identify specific groups of people who exhibit the characteristics of the social process or phenomenon under study. For example, a researcher may be seeking to interview people who have recently been bereaved; another researcher may be seeking people who have experienced long-term unemployment and suffer from chronic asthma. Sometimes researchers try to find people who typify the characteristics they are looking for. This is known as an 'ideal type'.

Occasionally it is useful to deliberately include people who exhibit the required characteristics in the extreme. Close examination of extreme cases can sometimes be very illuminating when trying to formulate a theory.

Another sampling technique commonly used in research is 'snowballing'. Snowballing occurs when one respondent supplies you with the names of other individuals in a like position, who may also be interested in talking to you. Snowballing is particularly useful when trying to reach individuals with rare or socially undesirable characteristics.

If a researcher wishes to develop a theory from her/his research, a 'theoretical sampling' technique may be used. The idea is that the researcher selects the subjects, collates and analyses the data to produce an initial theory which is then used to guide further sampling and data collection from which further theory is developed.

All these methods raise issues about the degree to which findings can be generalised or achieve transferability. Readers planning to use qualitative methods should refer to Chapter 6 in *Research Approaches in Primary Care*, which describes data collection by observation and discusses questions of external validity in qualitative research.

Exercise 2

This is an opportunity to review your learning from the first part of this chapter. Read the extract below from a journal article 'National asthma survey reveals continuing morbidity'.

National asthma survey reveals continuing morbidity

(*Prescriber, 19 March 1996*)

'A preliminary analysis of a survey of 44,177 people with asthma has revealed that for many the condition causes frequent symptoms and substantially interferes with daily life. There is also a trend for older people with asthma to experience more problems. More information about treatment was seen by many as the best way to improve care.

The Impact of Asthma Survey was conducted by Gallup on behalf of the National Asthma Campaign with funding from Allen & Hanburys. Questionnaires were given to people with asthma via surgeries, pharmacies, retail outlets, the media and direct mailing in the autumn of 1995; the respondents were therefore self-selected and may not be representative of the population with asthma.

Asthma symptoms were experienced on most days or daily by 41% of survey respondents, ranging from 18% of the under-11s to 55% of pensioners. Waking every night with wheeze, cough or breathlessness was reported by 13% and 43% say they are woken by symptoms at least once a week.

About 20% consider that asthma dominates their life, ranging from 17% in children to 37% in the over-60s; over 40% of each age group say the condition has a moderate impact on their quality of life.'

Now answer the following questions.

1.   How was the sample selected for this survey?
2.   Did the researchers use random or non-random sampling methods?
3.   What are the advantages of their approach?
4.   What are the disadvantages of this approach?

5. The sample size was 44 177. Why was the sample size so large and was this necessary?

Sample size and the power of research

In the previous section, we looked at methods of sampling. Now we want to turn to another aspect of sampling: how big a sample needs to be in quantitative research to enable a study to have sufficient 'power' to do the job of testing a hypothesis. While this discussion will necessarily take us into the realm of statistics, we will keep the 'number-crunching' to a minimum: what is important is that you understand the concepts (and know a friendly statistician!).

At first glance, many pieces of research seem to choose a sample size merely on the basis of what 'looks' about right, or perhaps simply for reasons of convenience: 10 seems a bit small, and 100 would be difficult to obtain, so 40 is a happy compromise! Unfortunately a lot of published research uses precisely this kind of logic. In the following section, we want to show you why using such reasoning could make your research worthless. Choosing the correct size of sample is not a matter of preference, it is a crucial element of the research process, without which you may well be spending months trying to investigate a problem with a tool which is either completely useless, or over-expensive in terms of time and other resources.

The truth is out there: hypotheses and samples

As we noted earlier, most (but not all) quantitative studies aim to test a hypothesis. A hypothesis is a kind of 'truth claim' about some aspect of the world: for instance, the attitudes of patients or the prevalence of a disease in a population. Research sets out to try to prove this truth claim right (or more properly, to disprove the null hypothesis – a truth claim phrased as a negative).

For example, let us think about the following hypothesis:

Levels of ill-health are affected by deprivation

and the related null hypothesis:

Levels of ill-health are not affected by deprivation

Let us imagine that we have this as our research hypothesis, and we are planning research to test it. We will undertake a trial, comparing groups of patients in a practice who are living in different socio-economic environments, to assess the extent of ill-health in these different groupings. Obviously the findings of a study – whilst interesting in themselves – only have value if they can be generalised. If we find an association, then we will want to do something to reduce ill-health (by reducing deprivation). So our study has to have external validity, that is, the capacity to be generalised beyond the subjects actually in the study.

The measurement of such generalisability of a study is done by statistical tests of inference. You will be familiar with some tests, such as the Chi-squared Test, the t-Test and tests of correlation (*see* p. 16). We need to understand that the purpose of these and other tests of statistical inference is to assess the extent to which the findings of a study can be accepted as valid for the population from which the study sample has been drawn. If the statistics we use suggest that the findings are 'true', then we can conclude that (within certain limits of probability) the study's findings can be generalised, and we can act on them (to improve nutrition among children under five years, for instance).

From common sense we can see that the larger the sample, the easier it is to be satisfied that it is representative of the population from which it is drawn: but how large does it need to be? To answer this question we need to consider further the possibilities that our findings may not reflect reality: that we have committed an error in our conclusions.

Type I and Type II errors

What any researcher wants is to be right! S/he wants to discover that there is an association between two variables: say, asthma and traffic pollution, *but only if such an association really exists*. If there is no such association, s/he wants her study to support the null hypothesis that the two are not related. (While the former may be more exciting, both are important findings.)

What no researcher wants is to be wrong! No one wants to find an association which does not really exist, or – just as importantly – *not* find an association which *does* exist. Both such situations can arise in any piece of research. The first (finding an association which is not really there) is called a 'Type I error'. It is the error of falsely rejecting a true null hypothesis. (This could also be called a 'false positive'. An example would be a study which rejects the null hypothesis that there is no association between ill-health and deprivation. The findings suggest such an association, but in reality, no such relationship exists.)

The second kind of error, called a Type II error, occurs when a study fails to find an association which really does exist. It is then a matter of wrongly accepting a false null hypothesis. (This is a 'false negative': using the ill-health and deprivation example again, we conduct a study and find no association, missing one which really does exist.)

Both types of error are serious. Both have consequences: imagine the money which might be spent on reducing traffic pollution, and all the time it does not really affect asthma (a Type I error). Or imagine allowing traffic pollution to continue, while it really is affecting children's health (a Type II error). Good research will minimise the chances of committing both Type I and Type II errors as far as possible, although they can never be ruled out absolutely.

Table 2.1   The null hypothesis (Ho), statistical significance and statistical power

		POPULATION	
Null hypothesis is		**False**	**True**
S		*Cell 1*	*Cell 2*
T	**False**	**Correct result**	**Type I error (alpha)**
U			
D		*Cell 3*	*Cell 4*
Y	**True**	**Type II error (beta)**	**Correct result**

Statistical significance and statistical power

For any piece of research that tries to make inferences from a sample to a population there are four possible outcomes: two are desirable, two render the research worthless. Table 2.1 shows these four possible outcomes.

Each cell in the table represents a possible relationship between the findings of the study and the 'real-life' situation in the population under investigation. (Of course, we cannot actually know the latter unless we surveyed the whole population: that is the reason we conduct studies which can be generalised through statistical inference.) Cells 1 and 4 represent desirable outcomes, whilst Cells 2 and 3 represent potential outcomes of a study which are undesirable and need to be minimised. We shall now consider the relationship between these possible outcomes and two concepts, that of 'statistical significance' and 'statistical power'. The former is well known by most researchers who use statistics, the latter less so. Let us look at these four outcomes, in relation to the study of ill-health and deprivation given as an example above.

Cell 1. The null hypothesis has been disproved by the results of the study, and there is support for a hypothesis which suggests an association between ill-health and deprivation. In 'reality' such an association does exist in the population. In this outcome, the study *is* reflecting the world outside the limits of the study and it is a 'correct' result (that is, the result is both statistically significant *and* clinically significant).

Cell 4. The results from the study support the null hypothesis: there is no association between ill-health and deprivation. This is the situation which pertains in the population, so once again in such circumstances the study reflects 'reality'. And once again, this is a 'correct' result which is neither statistically *nor* clinically significant.

Cell 2. In this cell the study results reject the null hypothesis, indicating some kind of association between the variables of deprivation and ill-health. However, these study results are false, because in the population from which we drew our sample the null hypothesis is actually true and there is no such association. This is a Type I error: the error of rejecting a true null hypothesis. The likelihood of committing a Type I error (finding an association which does not really exist) is known as the 'alpha' (α) value or the 'statistical significance' of a statistical test. Some of you may be familiar with α as p, the quoted level of significance of a test. The p value marks the probability of committing a Type I error; thus a p value of 0.05 (a widely used conventional level of significance) indicates a 5% – or one in 20 – chance of committing a Type I error. Cell 2 thus reflects an incorrect finding from a study, and the α value represents the likelihood of this occurring.

Cell 3. This cell similarly reflects an undesirable outcome of a study. Here a study supports the null hypothesis, implying that there is no association between ill-health and deprivation in the population under investigation. But in reality, the null hypothesis is false and there is an association which the study is missing. This mistake is the Type II error of accepting a false null hypothesis, and is the result of having a sample size which is too small to allow detection of the association by statistical tests at an acceptable level of significance (say $p = 0.05$). The likelihood of committing a Type II error is the 'beta' (β) value of a statistical test, and the value $(1-β)$ is the 'statistical power' of the test. Thus, the statistical power of a test is the likelihood of avoiding a Type II error. Conventionally, a value of 0.80 or 80% is the target value for statistical power, representing a likelihood that four times out of five a study will reject a false null hypothesis. Outcomes of studies which fall into Cell 3 are incorrect; β or its complement $(1-β)$ are the measures of the likelihood of such an outcome of a study.

All research should seek to avoid both Type I and Type II errors, which lead to incorrect inferences about the world beyond the study. In practice, there is a trade-off. Reducing the likelihood of committing a Type I error by increasing the level of significance at which one is willing to accept a positive finding reduces the statistical power of the test, thus increasing the possibility of a Type II error (missing an association which exists). Conversely, if a researcher makes it a priority to avoid committing a Type II error, it becomes more likely that a Type I error will occur (finding an association which does not exist). Now spend a few minutes doing this exercise to help you think about Type I and Type II errors in research.

Exercise 3

If we knew everything about the world, we would not need to do research. But we don't know everything, and research projects try to find out something more. With limited resources, we have to accept that sometimes (despite all efforts to conduct good research) our findings will be wrong. Use your judgement to decide in each of the four following pieces of research which poses the greater risk: a Type I or a Type II error, and why.

Research Study 1
A randomised controlled trial of a proven but expensive drug and an unproven cheap drug to treat HIV infection, to see if there is a difference in efficacy in controlling the disease.

Research Study 2
A study to test whether arrhythmias are more likely in patients taking a new anti-histamine prescribed for hayfever, compared with those already in use.

Research Study 3
A study to investigate the effect of training ambulance staff in defibrillator use on reducing numbers of 'dead-on-arrivals' after road traffic accidents.

Research Study 4
A survey of causes of deaths among white and ethnic minorities in the USA.

Calculating sample size

In the rest of this chapter, we will work through examples of the calculations needed to determine an appropriate sample size. First, we will look at descriptive studies (which do not test a hypothesis). Then we will consider issues of statistical significance and power in inferential studies.

Sample size in descriptive studies

Not all quantitative studies involve hypothesis testing, some studies merely seek to describe the phenomena under examination. Whereas hypothesis testing will involve comparing the characteristics of two or more groups, a descriptive survey may be concerned solely with describing the characteristics of a single group. The aim of this type of survey is often to obtain an accurate estimate of a particular figure, such as a mean or a proportion. For example, we may want to know how many times, in an average week, that a general practitioner sees patients newly presenting with asthma. In addition we may also want to know what proportion of these patients admit to smoking five or more cigarettes a day. In these circumstances, the aim is not to compare this figure with another group, but rather, to accurately reflect the real figure in the wider population.

To calculate the required sample size in this situation, there are certain things that we need to establish.

1. The level of certainty we require concerning the accuracy of the estimate of a mean or proportion. This is the 'level of significance'. Hence, a significance of 5%, or 0.05, indicates that we can be 95% certain that our estimate accurately reflects the true figure (but once in 20 times, the figure will be incorrect by chance). Alternatively, a 1% or 0.01 level gives us a 99% certainty that our data is correct. More certainty will require a larger sample size.

2. The degree of precision which we can accept. This is known as the 'confidence interval'. For example, a survey of a sample of patients indicates that 35% smoke.

Table 2.2   Precision (confidence intervals) and necessary sample sizes for a population with 35% smokers

Confidence interval	Sample size
+ or – 10%	88
+ or – 5%	350
+ or – 3%	971
+ or – 2%	2188
+ or – 1%	8750

Are we willing to accept that the figure for the wider population lies between 25 and 45% (a confidence interval of 10% either way), or do we want to be more precise, such that the confidence interval is 3% each way, and the true figure falls between 32 and 38%? As we can see from the above table, the smaller the confidence interval, the larger the sample must be.

We will look at how to calculate sample sizes for mean averages (for example, mean birth-weights) to supply different levels of precision (confidence intervals) in the following pages. In such studies, the confidence interval will depend upon the distribution of values in the sample: the more variability (as measured by the standard deviation) in the population, the greater the sample will need to be to supply a given confidence interval.

We also need to bear in mind the likely response rate. Allowance needs to be made for non-responses to a survey, so that this can be added on to the required sample size. For example, if our calculations indicate that we need a minimum sample size of 200, but we only expect a 70% response rate, then we will need to select an initial sample size of 267 to allow for possible non-response. It is particularly important to make an allowance for non-response when planning a longitudinal survey, when the same individuals will be repeatedly contacted over a period of time, since cumulative non-response can result in the final wave of the survey being too small to analyse.

Worked example 1: how large must a sample be to estimate the mean value of the population?

Suppose we wish to measure the number of times that the average patient with asthma consults her/his general practitioner for treatment.

The formula to calculate the sample size for a mean (or point) estimate is:

$$N = (SD/SE)^2$$

where N = the required sample size
        SD = the standard deviation
        SE = the standard error of the mean.

The SE (standard error) is calculated by deciding upon the accuracy level which you require. If, for instance, you wish your survey to produce a very accurate answer with only a small confidence interval, then you might decide that you want to be 95% confident that the mean average figure produced by your survey is no more than plus or minus two visits to the GP.

**If the significance level is 95%, then divide the confidence interval
by 1.96 to find the SE
If the significance level is 99%, then divide the confidence interval
by 2.56 to find the SE**

For example, if you thought that your survey might produce a mean estimate of 12.5 visits per year, then your confidence interval in this case would be 12.5 ± two visits. So the true range of visits in the population would range from 10.5 to 14.5 visits per year.

Now decide on your required significance level. If you decide on 95% (meaning that 19 times out of 20 the true population mean falls within the confidence limit of 10.5 and 14.5 visits), the standard error is calculated by dividing the confidence interval by 1.96. So, in this case, the standard error is 2 divided by 1.96 = 1.02.

The standard deviation could be estimated either by looking at some previous study or by carrying out a pilot study. Suppose that previous data showed that the standard deviation of the number of visits made to a GP in a year was 10, then we would input this into the formula as follows:

$$N = (SD/SE)^2$$
$$N = (10/1.02)^2$$
$$N = 9.8^2 = 96$$

If we are to be 95% confident that the answer achieved is correct ± two visits, then the required sample is 96.

Worked example 2: how large must a sample be to estimate a proportion/percentage?

Suppose that we were interested in finding out what percentage of the local patient population were satisfied with the service they had received from their GP over the previous 12 months. We want to carry out a survey, but of how many people?

Once again we need to know:

- the significance level (level of certainty)
- the confidence interval we are willing to accept, for example that our survey finding lies within plus or minus 5% of the population figure.

Assume that we decide that the precision with which we decide the proportion of respondents who say that they are satisfied with the service must be plus or minus 5%. This then is our confidence interval. To calculate the standard error, we divide the confidence interval by 1.96. In this case the standard error is $5/1.96 = 2.55$.

We also need to estimate the proportion which we expect to find who are satisfied. In order to estimate P (the estimated proportion) we should consult previous surveys or conduct a pilot. Assume, for the time being, that a similar survey carried out three years ago indicated that 70% of the respondents said they were satisfied. We then use the following formula:

$$N = \frac{P(100 - P)}{(SE)^2}$$

With P = 70% and SE = 2.55

$$N = \frac{70(100 - 70)}{(2.55)^2}$$

$$N = \frac{2100}{6.5}$$

$$N = 323$$

So, in order to be 95% confident that the true proportion of people saying they are satisfied lies within ± 5% of the answer, we will require a sample size of 323. This assumes that the likely answer is around 70%, with a range between 65% and 75%.

Of course, in real life, we often have absolutely no idea what the likely proportion is going to be. There may be no previous data and no time to carry out a pilot. In these circumstances, it is safer to assume the worst case scenario and assume that the proportion is likely to be 50%. This will allow for the largest possible sample size.

If we wished to use a 99% level of significance, so we might be 99% certain that our confidence parameters include the true figure, then we need to divide the confidence interval by 2.58. In this case, the standard error would be $5/2.58 = 1.94$. Using the formula above, we find that this would require a sample size of 664.

Exercise 4

Calculating sample sizes for descriptive surveys.

1. You want to conduct a survey of the average age of GPs in the UK:
    *   your significance level is 95%
    *   your acceptable confidence limit is plus or minus three years
    *   from previous work you estimate that the standard deviation is 13 years.

a)   Using the following formula to calculate sample sizes for a mean estimate, calculate the sample size: N = ...

$$N = (SD/SE)^2$$

(recalling that the SE is calculated as the confidence interval/1.96).

b)   What would the sample size need to be if the response rate to the survey is 70%?

N = ...

2.   You want to conduct a survey of the proportion of men over 65 who have cardiac symptoms:
   •   your significance level is 95%
   •   your acceptable confidence limit is plus or minus 2%
   •   from previous work you estimate that the proportion is about 20%.

a)   Using the following formula to calculate sample sizes for a proportion, calculate the sample size: N = ...

$$N = \frac{P(100 - P)}{(SE)^2}$$

b)   What would the sample size need to be if the response rate to the survey is 80%?

N = ...

Sample size in inferential studies

As we saw earlier in this chapter, studies which test hypotheses (seeking to generalise from a study to a population) need sufficient power to minimise the likelihood of Type I and Type II errors. Both statistical significance and statistical power are affected by sample size. The chances of gaining a statistically significant result will be increased by enlarging a study's sample. Similarly, the statistical power of a study is enhanced as sample size increases. Let us look at each of these aspects of inferential research in turn. You may wish to refer back to Table 2.1.

The statistical significance of a study

When a researcher uses a statistical test of inference, what s/he is doing is testing results against a gold standard. If the test gives a positive result (this is usually known as 'achieving statistical significance'), then s/he can be relatively satisfied that the results are 'true', and that the real-world situation is that discovered in the study (Cell 1 in Table 2.1). If the test does not give significant results (non-significant or NS), then s/he can be reasonably satisfied that the results reflect Cell 4, where no association has been found and no such association exists.

However, we can never be absolutely certain that we have a result which falls in Cells 1 or 4. Statistical significance represents the likelihood of committing a Type I error (Cell 2). Let us imagine that we have results suggesting an association between ill-health and deprivation, and a t-Test (a test to compare the results of two different groups) gives a value which indicates that at the 5% or 0.05 level of statistical significance, there is more ill-health among a group of high scorers on the Jarman Index of deprivation than among a group of low scorers.

What this means is that 95% of the time, we can be certain that this result reflects a true effect (Cell 1). Five per cent of the time, it is a chance result, following random associations in the sample we chose. If the t-Test value is higher, we might reach 1% or 0.01 significance. Now, only 1% of the time will the result be a chance association.

Tests of statistical significance are designed to account for sample size, thus the larger a sample, the 'easier' it is for results to reach significance. A study which compares two groups of 10 patients will have to demonstrate a much greater difference between the groups than a study with 1000 patients in each group. This is fair: the larger study is much more likely to be 'representative' of a population than the smaller one. To summarise: statistical significance is a measure of the likelihood that positive results reflect a real effect, and that the findings can be used to make conclusions about differences which really exist.

The statistical power of a study

Because of the way statistical tests are designed, as we have just seen, they build in a safety margin to avoid generalising false-positive results which could have disastrous or expensive consequences. But researchers who use small samples also run the risk of not being able to demonstrate differences or associations which really do exist. Thus they are in danger of committing a Type II error (Cell 3 in Table 2.1), of accepting a false null hypothesis. Such studies are 'under-powered', not possessing sufficient statistical power to detect the effects they set out to detect. Conventionally, the target is a power of 80% or 0.8, meaning that a study has an 80% likelihood of detecting a difference or association which really exists.

Examination of research undertaken in various fields of study suggests that many studies do not meet this 0.8 conventional target for power (Fox and Mathers 1997). What this means is that many studies have a much-reduced likelihood of being able to discern the effects which they set out to seek: a study with a power of 0.66 will only detect an effect two times out of three, while studies with a power of 0.5 or less will detect effects at levels less frequent than those achieved by tossing a coin. A non-significant finding of a study may thus simply reflect the inadequate power of the study to detect differences or associations at levels which are conventionally accepted as statistically significant.

In such situations one must ask the simple question of such research: 'Why did you bother, when your study had little chance of finding what you set out to find?'

Statistical power calculations can be undertaken after a study has been completed, to assess the likelihood of a study having discovered effects. More importantly, such calculations need to be undertaken prior to a study to avoid the wasteful consequences of under-powering (or of over-powering in which sample sizes are excessively large, leading to very high power, but higher than necessary study costs). Power is a function of three variables: sample size, the chosen level of statistical significance (α) and effect size. While calculation of power entails recourse to tables of values for these variables, the calculation is relatively straightforward in most cases.

Effect size and sample size

As was mentioned earlier, there is a trade-off between significance and power, because as one tries to reduce the chances of generating false-negative results, the likelihood of a false-positive result increases. Researchers need to decide which is more crucial, and set the significance level accordingly. In Exercise 3, you had to decide whether a Type I or Type II error was more serious, based on clinical and other criteria.

Fortunately, both statistical significance and power are increased by increasing sample size, so increasing sample size will reduce likelihoods of both Type I and Type II errors. However, that does not mean that researchers necessarily need to vastly increase the size of their samples, incurring greater expense in time and resources.

The other factor affecting the power of a study is the effect size (ES), which is under investigation in the study. This is a measure of 'how wrong the null hypothesis is'. For example, we might compare the efficacy of two bronchodilators for treating an asthma attack. The ES is the difference in efficacy between the two drugs. An effect size may be a difference between groups or the strength of an association between variables such as ill-health and deprivation.

If an ES is small, then many studies with small sample sizes are likely to be under-powered. But if an ES is large, then a relatively small-scale study could have sufficient power to identify the effect under investigation. It is sometimes possible to increase effect size (for example, by making more extreme comparisons, or undertaking a longer or more powerful intervention), but usually this is the intractable element in the equation, and accurate estimation of the effect size is essential for calculating power before a study begins, and hence the necessary sample size.

An effect size can be estimated in four ways:

*   from a review of literature or meta-analysis, which can suggest the size of ES which may be expected
*   by means of a pilot study, which can gather data from which the size of effect may be estimated
*   by making a decision about the smallest size of effect which it is worth identifying. To consider the example of two rival drugs, if we are willing to accept the two drugs as equivalent if there is no more than a 10% difference in their efficacy of treatment, then this effect size may be set, acknowledging that smaller effects will not be discernible

- as a last resort, one can use a 'guesstimate' as to whether an ES is 'small', 'medium' or 'large'. These definitions and values for 'small', 'medium' and 'large' effects are conventions. A 'medium' effect is defined as one which is 'visible to the naked eye' – in other words – which could be discerned from everyday experience without recourse to formal measurement. For example, the difference between male and female adult heights in the UK would be counted as a medium ES. Most effects encountered in biomedical and social research should be assumed to be small, unless there is a good reason to claim a medium effect, while a 'large' effect size would probably need to be defined as one which is so large that it hardly seems necessary to undertake research into something so well established. Cohen offers the example of the difference between the heights of 13- and 18-year-old girls as a 'large' effect.

A case study of statistical power: primary care research

Power calculations may be used as part of the critical appraisal of research papers. Unfortunately it is rare to see β values quoted for tests in research reports, and indeed often the results reported are inadequate to calculate effect sizes. Appraisals of various scientific subjects, including nursing, education, management and general practice research, have been undertaken by various authors.

Now read the extract from an article by Fox and Mathers (1997).

'To explore the power of general practice research, we analysed all the statistical tests reported in the British Journal of General Practice (BJGP) over a period of 18 months. Power was calculated for each test based on the reported sample size. This enabled calculation of the power of each quantitative study published during this period, to assess the adequacy of sample sizes to supply sufficient power.'

Method

All original research papers published in the *BJGP* during the period January 1994 to June 1995 inclusive were analysed in terms of the power of statistical tests reported. Qualitative papers were excluded, as were meta-analyses and articles which, although reporting quantitative data, did not report any formal statistical analysis even though in some instances such tests could have been undertaken. A further six papers were excluded because they did not use standard statistical tests for which power tables were available. This left 85 papers, involving 1422 tests for which power could be calculated using power tables. Power was calculated for each test following conventions of similar research into statistical power. Where adequate data were available (for example details of group means and standard deviations, or Chi-Square Test results) precise effect sizes could be calculated. Where this was not possible (in particular for results simply reported

Table 2.3   Power of studies (N = 85)

Power band	N	%
<0.25	2	2
0.26–0.49	19	22
0.50–0.79	27	32
0.80–0.96	21	25
⩾0.97	16	19

as 'non-significant') the following assumptions were made, all of which considerably over-estimate the power of the test:

- for significant results, the effect size was assumed to be 'medium', which, as noted earlier, means an effect 'visible to the naked eye'. Non-significant results were assumed to have a 'small' ES
- alpha values were set at the lowest possible conventional level of 0.05, and where a directional test was used, a one-tailed alpha was used (equivalent to two-tailed alpha of 0.1).

From the calculations of power for individual tests, a mean power for each paper was derived. This strategy has been adopted in other research into statistical power: what is reported is study power, rather than test-by-test power, and it offers an estimate of the quality of studies in terms of overall adequacy of statistical power.

Results

Eighty-five papers comprising 1422 tests were analysed. The median number of tests per paper was 12, with a minimum of one test and a maximum of 90. The median power of the 85 studies was 0.71, representing a slightly greater than two-thirds probability of rejecting null hypotheses. The proportions of tests in different power bands is summarised in Table 2.3. Of the 85 studies, 37 (44%) had power of at least 0.8, while 48 (56%) fell below this conventional target. The lowest power rating was 0.24, while 10 studies (12%) reached power values of 0.99 or more.

Unlike some earlier studies of statistical power, no attempt has been made to subdivide studies into those with large, medium and small effect sizes, partly because in a number of cases the effect sizes were probably over-estimated as 'medium', and because within a single paper many different variables with differing effect sizes might be under investigation.

Discussion

The results of this survey of general practice research published in the *BJGP* indicates somewhat higher power ratings than those reported for other disciplines, including nursing, psychology, education, management and some medical journals. However over half of the studies fall below the conventional figure of 0.8, and 25% have a power of 0.5 or less, suggesting a chance of gaining significant results poorer than that obtained by tossing a coin.

Scrutiny of the distribution of powers indicated bimodality. Of the papers meeting or exceeding the 0.8 target, 16 out of 37 had powers of more than 97%. Such high powers were achieved by the use of very large samples. Given that it is necessary to double the sample size to increase power from 0.8 to 0.97, it is reasonable to argue that as such the studies were over-powered, using sample sizes which were excessively expensive in terms of researcher time for data collection and analysis. In some cases these studies used pre-existing data sets and so this criticism is less pertinent; elsewhere, researchers may have devoted far greater efforts in terms of time and obtaining goodwill from subjects than may strictly have been necessary to achieve adequate power. The importance of pre-study calculations of necessary sample size to achieve statistical power of 0.8 or thereabouts is relevant both for those studies demonstrated to be under-powered and those for whom power is excessive.

Conclusions and recommendations

More than half of the quantitative papers published in the *BJGP* between January 1994 and June 1995 were 'under-powered'. This means that during the statistical analysis, there was a substantial risk of missing significant results. Twenty-five per cent of papers surveyed had a chance of gaining significant results (when there was a false null hypothesis) which were poorer than that obtained from tossing a coin. We would make the following recommendations concerning the use of statistical power analysis in general practice research:

- all primary care and general practice researchers should use power calculations to decide on the necessary sample size before starting research.

Furthermore, we would tactfully request that:

- editors should ask authors to report the value of each test statistic with the alpha and beta values as well as sample size, to enable readers to assess the power of a study
- all such values for non-significant results should also be reported.

Exercise 5

1. What was the average power of research in the papers surveyed?
2. What proportion of papers had too high a power, and why is this an issue?
3. What recommendations do Fox and Mathers suggest to writers of papers which report tests of statistical inference?

Table 2.4   Necessary sample sizes for common statistical tests

Test	Degrees of freedom	ES = small	ES = medium
t-Test		300 per group	50 per group
F-Test (ANOVA)	2	322 per group	64 per group
	3	274 per group	45 per group
	4	240 per group	49 per group
Chi-Square	1	785 total	87 total
	2	964 total	107 total
	3	1090 total	121 total
Pearson's correlation		618	68

Worked example: calculating the sample size in inferential studies

We will work through two examples of power calculations. These provide formulae for calculating power for Chi-Square and t-Tests, although when calculating sample sizes most people will refer to tables or use computer software (*see* Further reading and resources on p. 52). Table 2.4 gives some rough and ready figures for a range of simple tests, based on a power ($1-\beta$) value of 0.8 and a significance level of 0.05 (5%), for 'small' and 'medium' effect sizes. You may be surprised to see how large the samples may need to be. (NB The 'degree of freedom' (df) of a statistical test is an indicator of the number of categories into which respondents are sub-divided. An F-Test (analysis of variance) of three groups of subjects has df = 3–1 = 2; a Chi-Square Test with a 2×2 table (for example, men and women satisfied and dissatisfied with a GP) has df = 1. Refer to a statistical text for details of how to calculate dfs for different tests.)

Worked example: sample size for tests of contingency

Imagine a doctor wanted to set up a double-blind trial of a new drug, to compare mortality after a stroke among patients using the new drug or a placebo.

1. Measure: death from any cause within one year of first treatment.
2. Analysis: comparison of proportion of deaths amongst new drug and placebo patients, using Chi-Square at $\alpha = 5\%$ significance.
3. Standard treatment: 90% expected to survive at least one year on placebo.
4. Power required: if the new drug can halve the mortality (reduce deaths from 10% to 5%), this should be detected 90% of time (power = 0.9, $\beta = 0.1$).

In summary:

p_1 = proportion of successes on standard treatment = 90%
p_2 = proportion of successes on the new drug which indicate it as more effective = 95%
α = 0.05
β = 0.1
K = constant which is a function of α and β (*see* Table 2.5).

Table 2.5   Values of K for sample size calculations

	β			
	0.5	0.2	0.1	0.05
0.1	2.7	6.2	8.6	10.8
0.05	3.8	7.9	10.5	13.0
0.02	5.4	10.0	13.0	15.8
0.01	6.6	11.7	14.9	17.8

The sample size for each group, N, is given by

$$N = \frac{[p_1(1-p_1) + p_2(1-p_2)] \times K}{(p_1-p_2)^2}$$

Look up the value of K for $\alpha = 0.05$ and $\beta = 0.1$ in Table 2.5.

Thus,

$$N = \frac{[(0.9 \times 0.1) + (0.95 \times 0.05)] \times 10.5}{(0.95 \times 0.9)^2}$$

$$N = 578 \text{ patients in each group (total} = 1156)$$

Note that here the difference between p_1 (success rate of placebo) and p_2 (success rate of the new drug) was very small. In other words, it was a very small effect size. Also the power required was very high (90%). If the effect size was larger or the power required was lower, the sample size would be substantially smaller.

Worked example: sample size for test of differences (t-Test)

A clinical trial tests the effect on neonatal hypocalcaemia of giving Supplement A to pregnant women. Women are randomised and given either placebo or Supplement A.

1. Measure: serum calcium level of baby one week postnatally.
2. Analysis: comparisons of difference between two groups of babies using an independent-samples t-Test at 5% significance ($\alpha = 0.05$).
3. Serum calcium in babies of untreated women 9.0 mg/100 ml, standard deviation (σ) 1.8 mg/100 ml.
4. Study should detect clinically relevant increase in serum calcium of 0.05 mg/100 ml, 80% of the time ($\beta = 0.2$).

In summary:

μ = mean serum calcium level = 9.0 mg/100 ml

σ = standard deviation = 1.8 mg/100 ml

d = difference in means $\mu_1-\mu_2$ = 0.5 mg/100 ml

α = 0.05

β = 0.2

The number of patients required in each group is given by

$$N = \frac{2 \times \sigma^2 \times K}{(\mu_1-\mu_2)^2}$$

where K is taken from Table 2.4

$$N = \frac{2 \times (1.8)^2 \times 7.9}{(0.5)^2}$$

$$N = 205$$

Exercise 6

Calculating sample size for inferential statistics.

1. A randomised controlled trial is carried out to investigate whether aspirin can prevent pregnancy-induced hypertension and pre-eclamptic toxaemia in women at high risk (Schiff *et al.* 1989):

- measure: trial and placebo group: develop or did not develop hypertension
- analysis: Chi-Square Test at 5% significance
- current situation: 30% of women develop hypertension
- power required: clinically useful reduction by one-third to 20% should be detected with 80% (β = 0.2) power.

    Calculate the necessary sample size.

2. A double-blind placebo-controlled trial is designed to test the effect of adding salmeterol to current treatment with inhaled corticosteroids in asthma sufferers who control their dosage according to a management plan (Wilding *et al.* 1997):

- measure: dosage of corticosteroids after six months of trial
- analysis: comparison of differences in dosage between test and placebo group using t-Test at α = 5% significance
- current level: mean dosage of corticosteroids 700 micrograms (standard deviation σ = 200 micrograms)
- power required to detect clinically relevant fall in dosage of 100 micrograms is 80% (β = 0.2).

    Calculate the number of subjects required in each treatment.

Summary

Key points to remember when deciding on sample selection are:

- try to use a random method where possible and remember that random does not mean haphazard
- random selection means that everybody in your sampling frame has an equal opportunity of being included in your study
- if you need to be able to generalise about small or minority groups and to compare those with larger groups, consider using disproportionate stratified sampling, but remember to re-weight the results afterwards if you wish to generalise from the whole sample.

Key points to remember when deciding on sample size are:

- a Type I error is the error of falsely rejecting a true null hypothesis
- the likelihood of committing a Type I error is known as alpha (α) and is equivalent to the *p* value of a test of significance. (Conventional levels for α are 0.05 (5%) or 0.01 (1%).)
- a Type II error is the error of failing to reject a false null hypothesis or wrongly accepting a false null hypothesis
- the likelihood of committing a Type II error is known as beta (β). (The conventional level of statistical power ($1-\beta$) is set at 0.8 or 80%.)
- there is a trade-off between committing a Type I error and a Type II error, but historically science has placed the emphasis on avoiding Type I errors
- increasing the sample size enables both α and β to be set at lower levels, and so will help reduce both Type I and Type II errors, but remember that it is costly and unethical to have too large a sample size
- to calculate statistical power, you need to estimate the effect size
- to estimate the sample size for a descriptive study in order to estimate a mean or a proportion, it is necessary to calculate the required confidence interval.

Answers to exercises

Exercise 1

1. Stratified random sample. The sample is stratified because the sample has been selected to ensure that two different groups are represented.
2. Disproportionate stratified random sample. This sample is stratified to ensure that patients from the two different groups are picked up, however the two groups are selected, so that they are equal in size and are not representative of the patient base.

3. Quota. The sample is not randomly selected, but the respondents are selected to meet certain criteria.
4. Convenience. The sample is not randomly selected and no quotas are applied.
5. Systematic random sample.
6. Cluster sample. The patients are selected only from certain wards.

Exercise 2

1. The researchers used a convenience sampling approach, i.e. they selected people on the basis that they were easy to access. Respondents were therefore self-selected.
2. The sampling method used was non-random.
3. The advantage of this approach was that they were able to obtain the views of a large number of people very quickly and easily with little expense.
4. Unfortunately the convenience sample approach means that the sample is not representative of the population of individuals with asthma. Because a large part of the survey is made up of people attending in surgery and pharmacies, the sample will tend to over-represent those individuals requiring the most treatment. It will also over-represent those individuals who are most interested in expressing their opinions.
5. The sample achieved was very large because it was self-selected, and therefore the researchers would have had little control over how many people participated. The sample is unnecessarily large. In order to achieve a statistically representative view of the asthmatic population, it would not be necessary to select such a large sample. This study demonstrates the point that large samples alone do not necessarily mean that the study can achieve representativeness. The only true way of achieving a representative sample is to use random sampling methods. Reflect on the sample size in this study as you now go on to study the second part of this chapter.

Exercise 3

1. Type II error of accepting a false null hypothesis. If the study shows no difference in efficacy, missing a difference which is present, an effective but expensive drug may be dropped because of its cost, making treatment of patients less effective.
2. Type I error of rejecting a true null hypothesis. If an effect (increased levels of arrhythmias) is found this may lead to a useful drug being abandoned.
3. Your answer will depend on your reasoning. You might suggest a Type I error is more serious: if the training actually makes no difference (a true null hypothesis) but a study shows it does, then the findings may lead to innovating a procedure which is expensive and has risks associated with it. Alternatively, you might say a Type II error is more serious: a study failed to discover a real reduction (a false null

hypothesis), so a useful procedure is not implemented and lives are lost. Your value perspective will affect which you see as more risky or costly (in an economic or humanistic sense).

4.   Neither. A survey does not test a hypothesis. However, if a direct comparison were being made, the answer would probably be that a Type II error was more serious. Race is a very sensitive issue in the USA. Missing a difference that existed (and was later discovered) could be both unjust and socially and politically catastrophic.

Exercise 4

1.a)   The sample size needs to be 72 GPs. This is calculated as follows using the formula:

$$N = (SD/SE)^2$$

In this case SD is 13. We can calculate the SE by dividing the confidence interval by 1.96. So the

$$SE = 3/1.96 = 1.53$$

Using the formula above:

$$N = (13/1.53)^2$$

$$N = 8.49^2 = 72$$

b)   If the response rate is 70%, you will need to recruit 103 subjects.

2.a)   The sample size needs to be 1537. This is calculated using the formula below.

$$N = \frac{P(100 - P)}{(SE)^2}$$

SE can be calculated by dividing the confidence interval by 1.96:

$$SE = 2/1.96 = 1.02$$

With

$$P = 20\% \text{ and } SE = 1.02$$

$$N = \frac{20(100-20)}{(1.02)^2}$$

$$N = \frac{20 \times 80}{1.04}$$

$$N = \frac{1600}{1.04} = 1537$$

b)   If the response rate is 80%, you will need to recruit 1921 subjects.

Exercise 5

1.   The average power was 0.71 or 71%.
2.   12%. It is important because these studies are thus more costly than necessary to achieve acceptable power.
3.   Researchers should do a power calculation to decide the necessary sample size before they begin their research. They should give α and β values for all tests, including those which are not statistically significant.

Exercise 6

1. p_1 = proportion developing hypertension on placebo = 0.3
      p_2 = proportion developing hypertension on placebo which we wish to detect = 0.2
      α = 0.05
      β = 0.2

$$N = \frac{p_1(1-p_1) + p_2(1-p_2)}{(p_1-p_2)^2} \times K$$

$$N = \frac{(0.3 \times 0.7) + (0.2 \times 0.8)}{(0.3-0.1)^2} \times 7.9$$

N = 293 patients in each group.

2.   difference $\mu_1 - \mu_2$ = 100 micrograms
      standard deviation σ = 200 micrograms
      α = 0.05
      β = 0.8

$$N = \frac{2 \times \sigma^2}{(\mu_1-\mu_2)^2} \times K$$

$$N = \frac{2 \times 200^2}{100^2} \times 7.9$$

N = 63 subjects in each group.

References

Fox N J and Mathers N J (1997) Empowering your research: statistical power in general practice research. *Family Practice.* **14**(4).

Schiff E, Peleg E, Goldenberg M *et al.* (1989) The use of aspirin to prevent pregnancy-induced hypertension and lower the ratio of thromboxane A2 to prostacyclin in relatively high-risk pregnancies. *NEJM.* **321**: 351–6.

Wilding P, Clark M, Coon J T *et al.* (1997) Effect of long-term treatment with salmeterol on asthma control: a double blind, randomised crossover study. *BMJ.* **314**: 1441–6.

Further reading and resources

For details of sampling techniques

Bland M (1995) *An Introduction to Medical Statistics* (2e). Oxford University Press, Oxford.

Clegg F (1982) *Simple Statistics: A Course Book for the Social Sciences.* Cambridge University Press, Cambridge.

Florey D du V (1993) Sample size for beginners. *BMJ.* **306**: 1181–4.

For details of power calculations

Campbell M J, Julious S A and Altman D G (1995) Estimating sample sizes for binary, ordered, categorical and continuous outcomes in two group comparisons. *BMJ.* **311**: 1145–8.

Cohen J (1977) *Statistical Power Analysis for the Behavioural Sciences.* Academic Press, New York.

Machin D and Campbell M J (1997) *Sample Size Tables for Clinical Studies.* Blackwell Science, Oxford.

The software package *nQuery Advisor* provides simple and efficient means of calculating power and sample size. It may be obtained from *Statistical Solutions* (8 South Bank, Crosse's Green, Cork, Republic of Ireland. Tel: 00 353 21 319629; fax: 00 353 21 319630; e-mail: sales@statsol.ie).

The software Epi Info also provides information on calculating sample sizes and can be obtained for little or no charge from a local public health department, an academic department of general practice, or from a local audit advisory group.

Studies of power in different scientific disciplines

Fox N J and Mathers N J (1997) Empowering your research: statistical power in general practice research. *Family Practice.* **14**(4).

Polit D F and Sherman R E (1990) Statistical power in nursing research. *Nursing Research.* **39**: 365–9.

Reed J F and Slaichert W (1981) Statistical proof in inconclusive 'negative' trials. *Archives of Internal Medicine.* **141**: 1307–10.

CHAPTER THREE

An introduction to using SPSS

Michael Hewitt

Introduction

Introductory material on SPSS for Windows is presented in the following section. The core material of the chapter is presented in three sections, namely: *Summarising and presenting data*, *Testing hypotheses* and *Examining relationships*. Each one provides example data sets and step-by-step instructions of how to analyse the data. Screen shots of expected outputs are given.

The aim of part two of the chapter is to provide a practical introduction to SPSS for Windows. As with part one, after completion you will be able to:

* enter and save data
* produce summary statistics and charts
* analyse data sets.

SPSS for Windows: an introduction

SPSS for Windows is a software package for statistical data analysis. It was originally developed for the social sciences, hence the acronym SPSS (Statistical Package for the Social Sciences) but is now used in many areas of scientific study.

This brief section serves as an introduction to the package and will show you how to start the software, enter and save data. It is written as a step-by-step, interactive exercise, which you can follow if you have access to SPSS for Windows.

Starting SPSS for Windows

The Windows Program Manager is used to organise and run software packages. An example of a Program Manager window is shown in Figure 3.1 (the contents of your Program Manager window may differ from the one below).

To start SPSS for Windows:

• **double-click** with the left mouse button on the SPSS icon

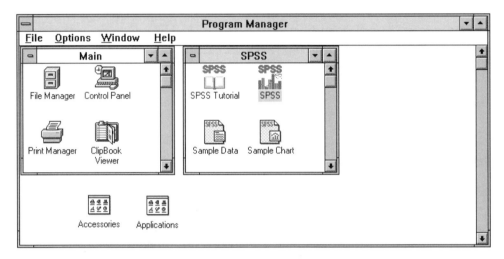

Figure 3.1 Windows Program Manager.

After double-clicking on the SPSS icon, the SPSS screen will appear (Figure 3.2).

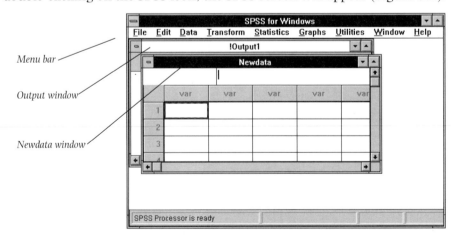

Figure 3.2 SPSS for Windows.[1]

[1] Screen shots from SPSS for Windows Version 6.1.3 are shown throughout this chapter with kind permission of SPSS Inc.

The **menu bar** displays the names of the menus that are available to you. When you click on a menu name, for example File, a list of commands is displayed. The File menu provides options for opening a file, saving a file, printing etc. Other commonly used menus and options are: Edit (to cut, copy or paste data), Statistics (to analyse data, for example summary statistics, correlation etc.), Graphs (to present data graphically, for example bar chart, histogram etc.), Window (to move from the Output window to the Newdata window, see below) and Help (including Help Contents, SPSS Tutorial, SPSS Glossary etc.).

The **Output window** is where SPSS displays the statistics and reports from the analysis of your data.

The **Newdata window** comprises a matrix of rows and columns similar to a spreadsheet. The rows represent individual cases (observations) and the columns represent variables.[2] A single cell is an intersection of a case and a variable, for example the height of person x.

Entering data

When you start SPSS you are automatically placed in the Newdata window. The active cell in the window has a heavy black border around it, indicating that any data you type will be entered into that cell. You can move around the Newdata window by using the arrow keys ($\leftarrow$, $\uparrow$, $\rightarrow$, $\downarrow$), or by clicking on cells with the mouse.

Table 3.1 presents some patient data that we can enter into SPSS. For each patient we have collected the following data from their medical notes: gender, age and blood group. The data have already been coded[3] by a researcher,

where for Gender: 1 = female, 2 = male
and for Blood group: 1 = A, 2 = AB, 3 = B, 4 = O

To enter the data into SPSS follow these instructions:

Starting with the black border in the top left cell of the Newdata window, type in the first value shown above under the column heading Gender, i.e. type 1 and press the enter key. The value is placed in the cell and the black border moves down to the next cell. Type in the other nine values, remembering to press the enter key after each one. Your Newdata window should now look like Figure 3.3.

---

[2] A variable is basically anything that can assume different values that are observed and recorded in research, e.g. height, weight, gender.
[3] Coding is the process whereby words or categories of a variable are changed into numbers so the computer can make statistical/numerical sense of the data (e.g. the variable Gender comprises the categories Female and Male and has been coded so that Female = 1 and Male = 2).

Table 3.1   Patient data

Gender	Age	Blood group
1	21	1
2	39	4
2	43	4
1	55	4
1	26	3
1	19	3
2	65	1
2	41	1
1	61	2
1	50	4

	Newdata			
	var00001	var	var	var
1	**1.00**			
2	**2.00**			
3	**2.00**			
4	**1.00**			
5	**1.00**			
6	**1.00**			
7	**2.00**			
8	**2.00**			
9	**1.00**			
10	**1.00**			

Figure 3.3   Newdata.

Now move the cursor to the top of the second column and type in the second column of data, Age, and then move to the top of the third column and enter the the third column of data, Blood group. If you make any mistakes during data entry, simply type over the entry and press the enter key.

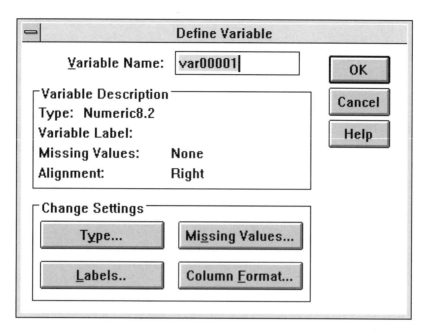

Figure 3.4　Define Variable.

Defining the variables

At the moment the first column is labelled **var00001**. This can be relabelled to show the name of the variable. We can also say more about the type of variable we are dealing with (for example, are the values numbers with or without a decimal place) and record the coding scheme we have used. This process is known as defining the variable and is described below:

* double-click the first grey column heading (currently labelled **var00001**). The **Define Variable** dialogue box appears (Figure 3.4).

We will amend the information about this variable in three ways:

1. Enter the name of the variable.
    * type the new name **gender** in the **Variable Name** box
    Variable names (column headings) can be no longer than eight characters and should not contain spaces (i.e. the name 'gender of patient' would not be allowed).
2. Change the number of decimal places.
    In the **Variable Description** box above, the Type of the variable is defined as Numeric8.2. This means that the column will accept numeric data with two

decimal places and display a maximum of eight digits for each number. This definition is fine for numbers that require this precision, e.g. height of patients in metres such as 1.65, 1.82. However, our data for the gender column requires less precision and can be accommodated in a column with no decimal places, i.e. whole numbers. This is done as follows:

• click on the **Type** button in the **Change Settings** box
• click in the **Decimal Places** box and type **0**.

Before clicking on the **Continue** button, examine the range of data types that are available. The Comma, Dot and Scientific Notation options provide for numeric data in different formats. The Date option allows calendar dates to be entered, e.g. 24-05-95. The Dollar and Custom currency options provide for currency data, e.g. £24.99. The String option is for uncoded text, e.g. 'The patient thanked staff for ...'

To return to the **Define Variable** box:

• click on **Continue**, then **OK**.

3. Enter labels.

Finally we can enter the coding scheme that we have used for this variable. This is important for two main reasons. First, it provides us with a permanent record of the scheme. Second, it makes interpretation of later analysis much easier as the codes and their meanings are given in full. To enter labels:

• click on **Labels** in the **Change Settings** box.

There are two parts to labelling. First we can label the variable itself. This allows us to give a more descriptive label than that given for the column heading. For example:

• in the **Variable label** box, type **gender of patient**.

The second part of the labelling exercise is to record the coding scheme used for the variable:

• click in the **Value** box and type **1**
• click in the **Value label** box and type **Female**
• click on the **Add** button
• click in the **Value** box and type **2**
• click in the **Value label** box and type **Male**
• click on the **Add** button
• click on **Continue,** then **OK**.

Define the other two variables, Age and Blood group. For the variable Age use **age** for the column heading; change the Type to **Numeric8.0**; and label the variable as 'Age of patient'. No value labels are required for the variable.

For the variable Blood Group use **bloodgp** for the column heading; change the Type to **Numeric8.0**; label the variable as 'Blood group of patient' and label the values as shown in Table 3.2.

The Newdata window should now look like Figure 3.5.

Table 3.2   Labels for the variable bloodgp

Value	Value label
1	A
2	AB
3	B
4	O

Newdata

	gender	age	bloodgp	var
1	1	21	1	
2	2	39	4	
3	2	43	4	
4	1	55	4	
5	1	26	3	
6	1	19	3	
7	2	65	1	
8	2	41	1	
9	1	61	2	
10	1	50	4	

Figure 3.5   Newdata.

Once we have typed data in to the Newdata window and defined the variables, it is important to save the data on your computer:

- click on the **File** menu
- click on **Save Data**
- type **pat_data** in the **File Name** box
- click on **OK**.

SPSS adds the extension **.sav** to the end of your filename, which helps in recognising data files in future sessions. The data is ready to be analysed. Examples of analysis using this and other data are shown in the next three sections.

Help

SPSS includes a comprehensive 'online' help system. The **<u>Help</u>** menu provides different kinds of help, e.g. 'Search for help on...', SPSS Tutorial and SPSS Glossary.

The 'Search for help on...' option provides help on a number of topics arranged in alphabetical order. Users can either scroll down the list and select topics or type in a search term. For example, suppose we wanted help on defining variables:

- click on the **<u>Help</u>** menu and select the 'Searching for help on...' option
- type in **defining variables** ('defining variables' is a recognised help subject and becomes highlighted)
- click on the **Show topics** button (this reveals the topics available in the lower half of the screen – shown in Figure 3.6)
- select the topic of interest and click on the **Go To** button for the on-screen help.

Help is also available as you work through tasks in SPSS. Note, for example, when defining variables in Figure 3.4 a Help button is available for selection. Clicking on the button takes you to the Help screen associated with that task.

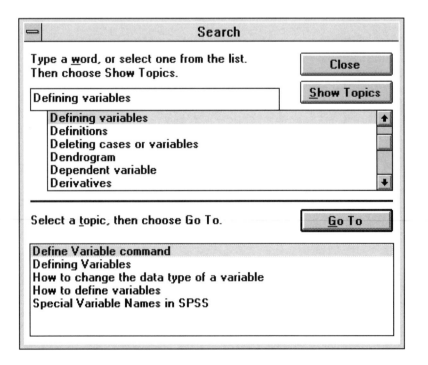

Figure 3.6   Search.

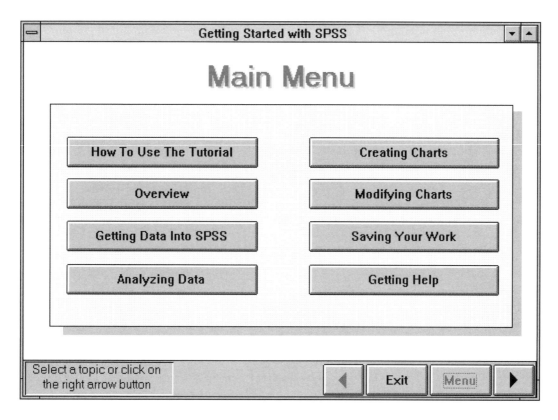

Figure 3.7   Tutorial Main Menu.

Experiment further with the Help system. For example, try the SPSS Tutorial – the opening screen is shown in Figure 3.7.

At any time you may want to exit SPSS. This is achieved with the following menu command:

• click on the **File** menu, then on **Exit**.

Summary

This section has introduced you to SPSS and has covered the first steps in using the package to analyse your data. This has included entering data, defining variables, saving data and using the Help system. It has also provided definitions of some of the key terminology used when analysing data. The following sections build on this work and introduce you to further features of the package.

Summarising and presenting data

The first step in any statistical analysis is summarising and presenting data. A simple summary statistic or graph will give you an immediate impression of the data you have collected. They also give a valuable check on any erroneous data that may have been entered by mistake and any missing data points.

Before we consider some methods used for summarising and presenting data, we need to consider the different types of data. These are: nominal, ordinal, and interval and ratio.

Nominal data: the observations are classified into categories that are different in character and cannot be measured or ordered. For example, gender, hair colour, blood group.

Ordinal data: the observations are classified into categories that can be ordered in an ascending series. For example, severity of an illness may be categorised as mild, moderate or severe.

Interval and ratio data: the observations are scores on a scale where the difference between scores is numerically equal. For example, height, weight.

The different types of data are important when considering the statistical analysis. The type of data determines the type of statistic that is appropriate for analysis. For further discussion of this topic, refer to Chapter 1 *An introduction to using statistics*.

Summarising data

Summary statistics include: the measures of location, for example mean, mode and median; and the measures of dispersion, for example range, interquartile range and standard deviation.

Summary statistics: measures of location

These give an idea of the position of an 'average' value on a particular scale of measurement.

The **mean** is the sum of all data points (observations or cases) divided by the number of data points, for example 7, 3, 11, 12, 9, 14, then the mean is 56/6 = 9.3.

The **median** is the middle value of a set of observations ranked in order (or the average of the two central numbers when there is an even number of observations), for example 14, 9, 17, 21, 7, 18, 16, 22. When ranked in order of size these are 7, 9, 14, 16, 17, 18, 21, 22. There are eight scores, so the median is the average of the fourth and fifth scores: (16+17)/2 = 16.5.

By obtaining the median you know that half of the observations have values that are smaller than the median, and the other half have values larger than the median. You can find values that split the sample in other ways. For example, you can find the value below which fall 25% of the data values. Such values are called 'percentiles', since they tell you the percentage of cases with values below and above them. For example, 25% of cases will have values smaller than the 25th percentile and 75% of cases will have values larger than the 25th percentile. The median is known as the 50th percentile, since 50% of cases have values less than the median and 50% have values greater than the median.

The **mode** is the most common value of a set of observations, for example 5, 2, 3, 4, 5, 6, 5, then the mode is 5.

Summary statistics: measures of dispersion

These are ways of describing the variability of data and include the range, interquartile range and standard deviation.

The **range** is the difference between the largest and smallest observations, for example 19, 21, 22, 22, 25, 27, 28, 42, then the range is $42-19 = 23$. A large value for the range tells you that the largest and smallest values differ substantially. It doesn't tell you about the variability of the values between the smallest and largest. A better measure of variability is the **interquartile range**. This is the difference between the 75th and 25th percentile values (see above).

One of the most commonly used measures of variability is called the **standard deviation**. It indicates the extent to which the scores (values) deviate from the mean score. It is defined as the average deviation from the mean.

Presenting data

Data presentation techniques include: bar charts, histograms, and frequency tables.

Data presentation: frequency table

A frequency table is a simple and effective way of presenting data. It is particularly suitable when observations fall into one of a number of different categories (nominal data). An example is shown in Table 3.3.

Table 3.3   Frequency table of blood groups

Group	No. of patients
O	56
A	31
B	18
AB	15
Total	120

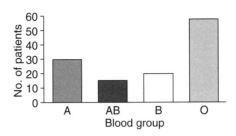

Figure 3.8   Bar chart of blood groups.

The first column shows the possible categories that the observations could take and the second column shows the frequency with which each category occurs. This is known as a 'frequency distribution'.

Data presentation: bar chart

A bar chart displays the frequency count for each category of a frequency distribution. Figure 3.8 shows the number of patients in each of the blood groups.

Data presentation: histogram

Histograms are similar to bar charts except that each bar represents a range of values. For example, a single bar may represent all the patients in Figure 3.8 with a haemoglobin percentage between 30 and 39. The midpoint, i.e. 34.5, is used to label the bar. A histogram of the haemoglobin data is shown in Figure 3.9.

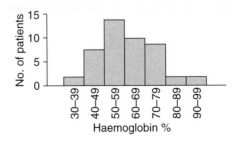

Figure 3.9   Histogram of haemoglobin %.

Table 3.4   Haemoglobin data

Haemoglobin %	Frequency (no. of patients)
30–39	2
40–49	7
50–59	14
60–69	10
70–79	8
80–89	2
90–99	2

Table 3.4 shows the number of patients with various percentage haemoglobin counts.

Exercise 1

This exercise explains how to summarise and present data using SPSS. The file created in the previous section **pat_data.sav** is used to demonstrate the main features of the package.

Load the file into SPSS via the **File** menu, followed by **Open** then **Data...**

1. Compute summary statistics for **age:**
    *   menu commands: **<u>S</u>tatistics** ⇒ **S<u>u</u>mmarize** ⇒ **<u>D</u>escriptives**...
    *   click on the variable **age**
    *   click on the arrowhead to move the variable to the right-hand box
    *   click on **OK**
    *   inspect the output window.

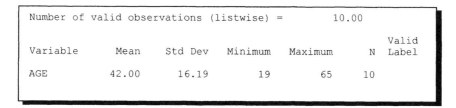

```
Number of valid observations (listwise) =        10.00

                                                    Valid
Variable     Mean     Std Dev   Minimum   Maximum   N   Label

AGE          42.00    16.19         19        65    10
```

2. Generate a frequency table for **bloodgp:**
    *   menu commands: **<u>S</u>tatistics** ⇒ **S<u>u</u>mmarize** ⇒ **<u>F</u>requencies**...
    *   click on the variable **bloodgp** in the left-hand box
    *   click on the arrowhead to move the variable to the right-hand box
    *   click on the button labelled **<u>S</u>tatistics**...
    *   locate the statistics grouped under the heading **Central tendency** and click on **Mode** (the box should be checked with a cross)
    *   click on **Continue**
    *   click on **OK**
    *   inspect the output window.

```
BLOODGP     Blood Group
                                                            Valid      Cum
   Value Label                    Value   Frequency   Percent   Percent   Percent

   A                                1          3       30.0      30.0      30.0
   AB                               2          1       10.0      10.0      40.0
   B                                3          2       20.0      20.0      60.0
   O                                4          4       40.0      40.0     100.0
                                                       -------   -------   -------
                                  Total       10      100.0     100.0

   Mode           4.000

   Valid cases      10     Missing cases      0
```

3.   Generate a bar chart for **bloodgp**:
     - menu commands: **Graphs** ⇒ **Bar**...
     - click on **Simple** and then on the button labelled **Define**
     - click on the variable **bloodgp**
     - click on the arrowhead next to the label **Category Axis**: to move the variable into the box. Check that Bars Represent <u>N</u> of Cases
     - click on **OK**
     - inspect the chart
     - click on the button labelled **Discard** when done.

Using similar techniques, generate a histogram of **age**.

Testing hypotheses

Introduction

One of the most important aspects of statistics is that concerned with making inferences or generalisations about a particular population on the basis of a sample drawn from that population. An assumption about the population is called a 'statistical hypothesis'.

The hypothesis we are trying to test is called the 'null' hypothesis (denoted H_0). The null hypothesis is the frame of reference against which you will judge your sample results. A contrary assumption is called the 'alternative' hypothesis (denoted H_1); this claims that the results differ from the frame of reference in a real or significant manner.

Hypotheses are best described by examples. Suppose we have a new drug to treat depression, drug x, and we want to discover whether it is more effective than an existing drug, drug y. The simplest hypothesis to test is that there is no difference in effectiveness between drug x and drug y. This would be the null hypothesis; it postulates the state of no difference. The alternative hypothesis would be that there is a difference in effectiveness between the two drugs.

We use appropriate experimental methods to gather evidence and then try to decide whether or not the null hypothesis is likely to be true. If the evidence is inconsistent with the null hypothesis then it is 'rejected'. If the evidence from the sample is consistent with the hypothesis then it is 'accepted'. The procedure we adopt in investigating the evidence is a 'statistical test'.

The result of a test is a decision to choose either H_0 or H_1. Such a decision is subject to uncertainty or error. Because of this the result is expressed as a probability (the p value).

There are numerous statistical tests available for analysing the significance of data. The selection of the appropriate test depends on the nature of the data to be analysed.

Two broad categories of tests have been developed and are referred to as 'parametric' and 'non-parametric' tests. Parametric tests are generally considered to be more powerful than non-parametric tests because they take into account more information about differences in scores. In general, parametric tests should only be used if your data fit the following specifications:

- interval or ratio data
- scores are normally distributed
- the two sets of scores have the same variance.

A detailed examination of these points is beyond the scope of this chapter. Interested readers can refer to statistics textbooks listed in *Further reading* on p. 80. Below, however, are some of the major tests, with a brief description of the appropriate data for each one. In each case analysis of the data is shown using SPSS. The data sets are examples only; they are simply used to demonstrate the different features of the statistical software.

Parametric tests

Paired t-Test

The paired-samples t-Test is used to test if two related samples come from populations with the same mean. The related, or paired, samples often result from an experiment in which the same person is observed before and after an intervention.

Example: To investigate the effects of exercise on blood glucose level in diabetics, blood glucose concentration (mmol/l) was measured in patients before and after a period of exercise (Table 3.5).

Exercise 2

This exercise explains how to use SPSS to analyse paired data using the t-Test. The data set for the analysis is the blood glucose measurements.

First we need to enter the data. Start with a blank **Newdata** window. Add two column headings (fields), named **before** and **after**, and type in the data as shown in Table 3.5 (no need to have a column for patient number).

Table 3.5   Blood glucose data

Patient	Blood glucose before	Blood glucose after
1	15.3	9.2
2	16.7	10.3
3	17.0	8.8
4	14.2	12.3
5	16.5	11.0
6	17.9	8.8
7	16.3	8.4
8	17.3	9.9
9	15.8	10.3

1. Menu commands: **Statistics** ⇒ **Compare <u>M</u>eans** ⇒ **<u>P</u>aired-Samples T-Test...**
2. Click on the variable **after**. It appears in the **Variable 1** box below.
3. Click on the variable **before**. It appears in the **Variable 2** box below (look in the **Current Selections** box to check whether you have done this correctly).
4. Click on the arrowhead.
5. Click on **OK**.
6. Inspect the output window.

```
t-tests for Paired Samples

                 Number of         2-tail
Variable           pairs    Corr   Sig        Mean         SD      SE of Mean
------------------------------------------------------------------------------
AFTER                                        9.8889      1.247         .416
                    9     -.602   .086
BEFORE                                      16.3333      1.112         .371
------------------------------------------------------------------------------


         Paired Differences        |
   Mean        SD    SE of Mean    |     t-value          df      2-tail Sig
------------------------------------|-----------------------------------------
-6.4444      2.113      .704       |      -9.15            8           .000
95% CI (-8.069, -4.820)           |
```

The test statistic t has a value of –9.15 and p = 0.000 (2-Tail Sig).

Table 3.6   Zinc sulphate data

Normal treatment and zinc sulphate	Normal treatment only
33	40
34	63
52	57
46	45
45	34
69	26
47	45
51	56
44	73

Independent-samples t-Test

The independent-samples t-Test is used when two samples of subjects provide scores on a measure. The t-Test compares the means of the two samples.

Example: In a trial of zinc sulphate on wound healing, nine patients were given oral zinc therapy in addition to normal treatment. A further nine patients received only their normal treatment. The time taken for 'complete healing' (in days) was measured; the data are shown in Table 3.6.

Exercise 3

This exercise explains how to use SPSS to analyse independent-samples data using the t-Test. The data set for the analysis is the zinc sulphate data.

First we need to enter the data. Start with a blank **Newdata** window. Add two column headings (fields), named **healtime** (no decimal places) and **group** (no decimal places). Under the heading healtime type in the nine values in the left-hand column (normal treatment and zinc sulphate) from the table above, directly followed by the nine values in the right-hand column (normal treatment only). Under the column group type in nine **1s**, directly followed by nine **2s**. Save your data as **wound.sav**. Your window should look like Figure 3.10.

1. Menu commands: **Statistics** ⇒ **Compare Means** ⇒ **Independent-Sample T-Test...**
2. Put the variable healtime in the box labelled **Test Variables(s)**.
3. Put the variable group in the Grouping Variable: box.
4. Click on **Define Groups...** in the box next to Group 1 enter 1 and in the box next to Group 2 enter 2.
5. Click on **Continue**.

	healtime	group	
1	33	1	
2	34	1	
3	52	1	
4	46	1	
5	45	1	
6	69	1	
7	47	1	
8	51	1	
9	44	1	
10	40	2	
11	63	2	
12	57	2	

Figure 3.10   Newdata window with zinc sulphate data.

6.   Click on **OK**.
7.   Examine the output window.

```
    t-tests for Independent Samples of GROUP

                           Number
Variable                   of Cases      Mean        SD    SE of Mean
-------------------------------------------------------------------------
HEALTIME

GROUP 1                         9       46.7778    10.628      3.543
GROUP 2                         9       48.7778    14.797      4.932
-------------------------------------------------------------------------

        Mean Difference = -2.0000

        Levene's Test for Equality of Variances: F= 1.886  P= .189


     t-test for Equality of Means                                   95%
Variances  t-value      df   2-Tail Sig   SE of Diff       CI for Diff
-------------------------------------------------------------------------
Equal         -.33      16       .746        6.073    (-14.873, 10.873)
Unequal       -.33   14.52       .747        6.073    (-14.981, 10.981)
-------------------------------------------------------------------------
```

The test statistic t = –0.33 and p = 0.746 (2-Tail Sig).

Table 3.7   Anxiety score data

Patient	Anxiety score with drug	Anxiety score with placebo
1	11	19
2	11	18
3	19	22
4	14	17
5	17	19
6	11	12
7	23	22
8	15	14
9	8	7
10	19	11

Non-parametric tests

Wilcoxon Matched-Pairs Test

This is the non-parametric counterpart of the related samples t-Test.

Example: The following are anxiety scores for 10 patients each receiving a new drug and placebo in random order. Table 3.7 presents the data. The null hypothesis would be that there is no difference between the treatments.

Exercise 4

This exercise explains how to use SPSS to analyse paired data using the Wilcoxon Matched-Pairs Test. The data set for the analysis is the anxiety data shown in Table 3.7.

First we need to enter the data. Start with a blank **Newdata** window. Add two column headings (fields), named **drug** and **placebo**, and type in the data as shown in Table 3.7 (no need to have a column for patient number).

1. Menu commands: **<u>Statistics</u> ⇒ <u>N</u>onparametric Tests ⇒ 2 Re<u>l</u>ated Samples...**
2. Click on the variable **drug**. It appears in the **Variable 1** box below.
3. Click on the variable **placebo**. It appears in the **Variable 2** box below (look in the **Current Selections** box to check whether you have done this correctly).
4. Click on the arrowhead.
5. Check that the Wilcoxon box is selected in **Test Type**.
6. Click on **OK**.
7. Examine the output window.

```
- - - - - Wilcoxon Matched-Pairs Signed-Ranks Test

       DRUG
with PLACEBO


   Mean Rank    Sum of Ranks  Cases

        4.25          17.00      4  - Ranks  (PLACEBO LT DRUG)
        6.33          38.00      6  + Ranks  (PLACEBO GT DRUG)
                                 0  0 Ties   (PLACEBO EQ DRUG)
                                --
                                10    Total

       Z =   -1.0787          2-Tailed P =  .2807
```

The test statistic is the smaller of the two 'sum of ranks', i.e. = 17 and p = 0.2807.

Mann-Whitney U Test

This is the non-parametric counterpart of the independent-samples t-Test.

Example: The energy expenditure of lean and obese groups of female subjects were measured over a 24-hour period (Table 3.8).

Table 3.8   Energy expenditure data

Energy expenditure (MJ/day)	
Lean (N = 13)	**Obese (N = 9)**
6.13	8.79
7.05	9.19
7.48	9.21
7.48	9.68
7.53	9.69
7.58	9.97
7.90	11.51
8.08	11.85
8.09	12.79
8.11	
8.40	
10.15	
10.88	

Exercise 5

This exercise explains how to use SPSS to analyse independent-samples data using the Mann-Whitney U Test. The data set for the analysis is the energy expenditure data shown in Table 3.8.

First we need to enter the data. Start with a blank **Newdata** window. Add two column headings (fields), named **energy** (two decimal places) and **group** (no decimal places). Under the heading energy type in the 13 values in the left-hand column (lean) from the table above, directly followed by the nine values in the right-hand column (obese). Under the column group type in 13 **1s**, directly followed by nine **2s**. Save your data as **energy.sav**.

1. Menu commands: **Statistics** ⇒ **Nonparametric Tests** ⇒ **2 Independent Samples...**
2. Put the variable **energy** in the **Test Variable**: box.
3. Put the variable **group** in the **Grouping Variable**: box.
4. Click on **Define Groups...** in the box next to **Group 1** enter **1** and in the box next to **Group 2** enter **2**.
5. Click on **Continue**.
6. Check that **Mann-Whitney U** is selected.
7. Click on **OK**.
8. Examine the output window.

```
 - - - - - Mann-Whitney U - Wilcoxon Rank Sum W Test


ENERGY
  by GROUP


    Mean Rank    Sum of Ranks   Cases
         7.92          103.0       13   GROUP    =      1
        16.67          150.0        9   GROUP    =      2
                                   --
                                   22   Total

                              Exact**
         U            W     2*(One-Tailed P)        Z      2-Tailed P
        12.0        103.0         .0011         -3.1061        .0019

**This exact p-value is not corrected for ties.
```

The test statistic = 150 and p = 0.0019.

Contingency tables

The techniques introduced here involve data in the form of frequencies. In other words, they deal with the situation where we are counting the number of times a particular event occurs.

Table 3.9   Attendance data

Status	Attended	Did not attend	Total
Reminder	30	9	39
No reminder	15	6	21
Total	45	15	60

Example: To determine whether an appointment reminder system is associated with a decrease in the number of non-attendances at a health-screening clinic. The results for a random sample of people are shown in Table 3.9.

This is called a contingency table. This type of data is suited to analysis with the Chi-Square Test (denoted χ^2). The null hypothesis is that the outcome, i.e. whether patients attended or did not attend their appointments, is independent of the reminder status.

Exercise 6

This exercise explains how to use SPSS to analyse contingency table data using the Chi-Square Test. The data set for the analysis is the attendance data shown in Table 3.9.

First we need to enter the data. Start with a blank **Newdata** window. Add two column headings (fields), named **remind** (no decimal places, labels 1=yes, 2=no) and **attend** (no decimal places, labels 1=yes, 2=no). Under the heading **remind** type in 39 **1s** (the number of patients sent reminders), directly followed by 21 **2s** (the number of patients not sent reminders). Under the heading **attend** type in 30 **1s** (the number who were sent a reminder and attended), directly followed by nine **2s** (received a reminder but didn't attend), directly followed by 15 **1s** (no reminder and attended), directly followed by six **2s** (no reminder, didn't attend). Save your data as **attend.sav**.

1. Menu commands: **Statistics** $\Rightarrow$ **Summarize** $\Rightarrow$ **Crosstabs...**
2. Put the variable **remind** in the **Rows(s):** box.
3. Put the variable **attend** in the **Column(s):** box.
4. Click on **Statistics...** and select **Chi-Square**.
5. Click on **Continue**.
6. Click on **OK**.
7. Examine the output window.

```
REMIND   by   ATTEND

                       ATTEND           Page 1 of 1
              Count   |
                      |Yes        No
                      |
                      |        1|        2|  Row
REMIND        --------+---------+---------+  Total
                 1    |   30    |    9    |     39
   Yes               |         |         |   65.0
              +--------+---------+---------+
                 2    |   15    |    6    |     21
   No                |         |         |   35.0
              +--------+---------+---------+
              Column       45        15        60
              Total      75.0      25.0     100.0

       Chi-Square                  Value         DF         Significance
  ---------------------          -----------    ----        ------------

Pearson                            .21978        1            .63921
Continuity Correction              .02442        1            .87582
Likelihood Ratio                   .21697        1            .64136
Linear-by-Linear                   .21612        1            .64201
     Association
Fisher's Exact Test:
   One-Tail                                                   .43195
   Two-Tail                                                   .75680

Minimum Expected Frequency -     5.250

Number of Missing Observations:   0
```

The test statistic (Pearson) = 0.21978 and p = 0.63921.

Examining relationships

This section considers the relationships between two measures. If two measures are shown to be related then (a) the description of the data can be simplified and (b) further research can be undertaken to determine the mechanisms which cause the measures to be related. The method of correlation is presented.

Correlation

Correlation is a measure of the extent to which two measures, for example height and weight, are related. The statistical measure of relation (or association) is known as the 'correlation coefficient' (denoted by the symbol r). Its value lies between -1 and $+1$; a large negative r indicates a negative association (Figure 3.11, Panel A); a large positive

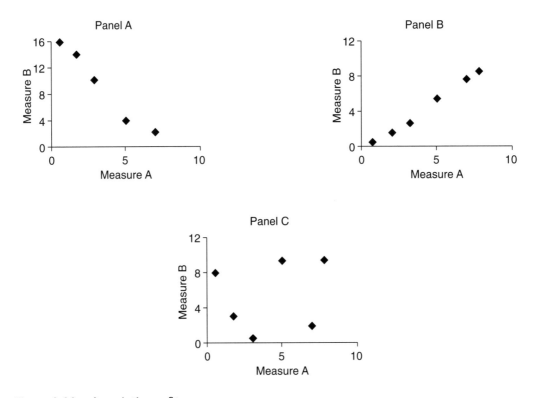

Figure 3.11   Associations of two measures.

r represents a positive association (Figure 3.11, Panel B); and a small r (either positive or negative) or $r = 0$ indicates little or no association at all (Figure 3.11, Panel C).

Example: Table 3.10 gives the results of a study in which 10 women had their haemoglobin level and packed cell volume (PCV) measured, together with their age.

Table 3.10   Haemoglobin and packed cell volume data

Patient	Hb	PCV	Age
1	11.1	35	20
2	10.7	45	22
3	12.4	47	25
4	14.0	50	28
5	13.1	31	28
6	10.5	30	31
7	9.6	25	32
8	12.5	33	35
9	13.5	35	38
10	13.9	40	40

Exercise 7

This exercise explains how to use SPSS to analyse the relationship between two measures using correlation. The data set for the analysis is the haemoglobin and packed cell volume data shown in Table 3.10.

First we need to enter the data. Start with a blank **Newdata** window. Add two column headings (fields), named **Hb** (one decimal place) and **PCV** (no decimal places). Type in the data in columns Hb and PCV as shown in Table 3.10.

1. Plot a scatter diagram to see the relationship between the two variables:
   - Menu commands: **Graphs** ⇒ **Scatter...**
   - Select the Simple type of plot and click on the **Define** button.
   - Put the variable **Hb** on the **Y Axis** and **PCV** on the **X Axis**.
   - Click on **OK**.
   - Examine the plot. Click on **Discard** when done.
2. Calculate Pearsons correlation coefficient.
   - Menu commands: **Statistics** ⇒ **Correlate** ⇒ **Bivariate...**
   - Put the variables **Hb** and **PCV** into the **Variables**: box.
   - Check that the **Pearson** box is selected.
   - Click on **OK**.
   - Examine the output window.

```
                        - -  Correlation Coefficients   - -

                  PCV           HB

    PCV            1.0000         .4725
                  (     9)      (     9)
                  P= .          P= .199

    HB              .4725        1.0000
                  (     9)      (     9)
                  P= .199       P= .


    (Coefficient / (Cases) / 2-tailed Significance)
```

The correlation coefficient, $r = 0.4725$ and $p = 0.199$.

Summary

This chapter has provided an introduction to the statistics package SPSS for Windows. Introductory material was presented in the first section, which included a step-by-step guide to entering data into the package. This was followed by three key sections, which described how to use SPSS for Windows to summarise and analyse different types of data sets. In each section, several illustrative examples were presented together with screen shots from the package showing expected outputs.

The chapter was written with the beginner in mind and to encourage use of the package rather than to produce an expert user. However, after working through the chapter it is likely that you have more questions now than when you started. Fortunately help is at hand from a number of sources. First, SPSS for Windows contains a comprehensive on-line Help system which should always be consulted should a question arise. Second, other manuals and textbooks are available, examples of which are listed in *Further reading* (below). Finally, there are many experienced users of SPSS for Windows in the field of health services research who may be willing and able to help.

When using a statistical package to analyse data we should not forget the wider context of the research process. This includes an appreciation of the research design, data collection, data analysis and interpretation of results. These aspects have not been discussed at length in this chapter. Further information can be found in other Trent Focus volumes in this series and textbooks of statistics, again examples of which are listed in *Further reading* (below).

This chapter has provided a practical step-by-step guide to SPSS for Windows for those new to the package. It is hoped that it has provided you with a firm foundation and confidence in using SPSS for Windows.

Further reading

Altman D G (1991) *Practical Statistics for Medical Research*. Chapman and Hall, London.

Bland M (1995) *An Introduction to Medical Statistics*. Oxford University Press, Oxford.

Brown R A and Swanson Beck J (1994) *Medical Statistics on Computers*. BMJ Publishing Group, London.

Puri B K (1996) *Statistics for the Health Sciences using SPSS*. Saunders, London.

Rowntree D (1991) *Statistics without Tears*. Penguin, London.

Swinscow T D V (1996) *Statistics at Square One* (9e) (revised by M J Campbell). BMJ Publishing Group, London.

CHAPTER FOUR

An introduction to using Epi Info

Michael Hewitt

Introduction

Introductory material on Epi Info is presented in the first section. The core material of the chapter is presented in three sections, namely: *Summarising and presenting data*, *Testing hypotheses* and *Examining relationships*. Each one provides example data sets and step-by-step instructions of how to analyse the data. Screen shots of expected outputs are given.

In working through this chapter it will become apparent that statistics packages cannot be divorced from the discipline of statistics. It is inevitable therefore, that the chapter includes coverage of some statistical concepts. It is hoped that this will aid learning rather than hinder you from working through the material.

The aim of this chapter is to provide a practical introduction to Epi Info. After working through the chapter you will be able to:

- enter and save data
- produce summary statistics and charts
- analyse data sets.

Epi Info: an introduction

Epi Info is a series of programmes produced jointly by the Centers for Disease Control and Prevention, USA and the World Health Organization. It was originally designed for the analysis of infectious disease outbreaks, but is flexible enough to be used as a general statistics package. Epi Info is available free of charge from the Centers for Disease Control and Prevention, USA.

This brief section serves as an introduction to the package and will show you how to start the software, enter and save data. It is written as a step-by-step, interactive exercise, which you can follow if you have access to Epi Info.

Starting Epi Info

Epi Info was developed before the days of the Windows environment. If you use a computer with Windows then you first need to exit from the Windows environment. This should take you to the 'c prompt': c:\>

At the 'c prompt' type: **cd \epi6** and press **enter**.
You will now see: **c:\EPI6>**
Now type: **EPI6** and press **enter**. The startup screen of the package should be displayed as shown in Figure 4.1.[1]

The top line of the screen is known as the **Menu Bar.** It displays the names of the menus that are available to you. The **File** menu shows options for opening a file, saving a file, printing etc. Other commonly used menus and options are: **Programs** menu (to enter and analyse data), **Edit** (to cut, copy or paste data) and **Manual** (to view the Help system).

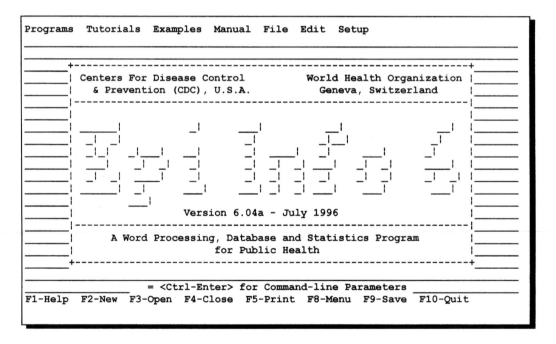

Figure 4.1   Epi Info startup screen.

---

[1] Screen shots from Epi Info Version 6.04a are shown throughout this chapter.

Table 4.1   Patient data

Gender group	Age	Blood
1	21	1
2	39	4
2	43	4
1	55	4
1	26	3
1	19	3
2	65	1
2	41	1
1	61	2
1	50	4

Menus and menu commands (options) are made available with the arrow keys ($\leftarrow$, $\uparrow$, $\rightarrow$, $\downarrow$) on the keyboard. To select an option from a menu press the Enter key.

Entering data

The process of entering data requires that we set up a 'questionnaire' file. This holds the variable[2] names of the data we have to analyse, for example gender, age, blood group, together with the type of data we are dealing with, for example numbers or text. The questionnaire file is converted into a 'record' file into which we type our data. The record file is then suitable for data analysis.

The data we are going to enter and analyse is shown in Table 4.1. For each patient we have collected the following data from their medical notes: gender, age and blood group. The data have already been coded[3] by a researcher,

where for Gender: 1 = female, 2 = male
and for Blood group: 1 = A, 2 = AB, 3 = B, 4 = O

Creating the 'questionnaire' file

Creating the questionnaire file is the first step in the data-analysis process. This is done in using the word processor 'EPED'.

*   start **EPED** by selecting it from the **Programs** menu

[2] A variable is basically anything that can assume different values that are observed and recorded in research, e.g. height, weight, gender.
[3] Coding is the process whereby words or categories of a variable are changed into numbers so the computer can make statistical/numerical sense of the data (e.g. the variable Gender comprises the categories Female and Male and has been coded so that Female = 1 and Male = 2).

The EPED screen (Figure 4.2) appears:

```
F1-Hlp F2-File F3-Epiaid F4-Txt F5-Print F6-Set F7-Find F8-Blk F9-Save F10-Done




1   UNTITLED                              EPED   321560      L1    C1   TXTInsInd
```

Figure 4.2   EPED screen.

Epi Info makes frequent use of the functions keys which lie across the top of your keyboard (F1, F2 etc.). Each key carries out a specific function or task. The keys and their associated tasks are shown along the top line of the screen. For the purpose of this chapter they are shown as <F1>, <F2> etc.

Follow the sequence of commands below to set up the questionnaire file. This involves typing in the variable names (known as 'fields') and information concerning the type of data, for example number or text. At the end of the sequence we will have a file into which we can type the patient data (from Table 4.1).

*   press **<F6>** to run the **SETUP** menu
*   press the **space bar** until the **QES** mode is selected on the right of the screen and press **Enter**
*   type the name of the first field **gender**
*   press **<Ctrl-QQ>** (that is, hold down the Ctrl key and type Q twice). A menu of field types appears on the screen 'Epi Info Questions'
*   select the second one on the list **##**. A box appears on the screen with the prompt 'How many digits before decimal point (0–10)?'
*   type **2** and press **Enter**. A box appears on the screen with the prompt 'How many decimal places (0–10)?'
*   enter **0** and press **Enter**. The screen shows **gender ##**.

To create the field **age**:

*   press **Enter** and type **age**
*   press **<Ctrl-QQ>** and select **##**
*   type **3** in response to prompt and press **Enter**
*   type **0** in response to second prompt and press **Enter**.

To create the field **bloodgp**:

*   press **Enter** and type **bloodgp** (without any spaces)
*   press **<Ctrl-QQ>** and select **##**
*   type **2** and press **Enter**
*   type **0** and press **Enter**.

The 'questionnaire' file has now been defined. To save the file press <F9> and enter the name **pat_data.qes** and press **Enter**. Finally press <F10> to exit the EPED.

Entering data into the 'record' file

From the Programs menu select Enter data. The Enter screen (Figure 4.3) appears:

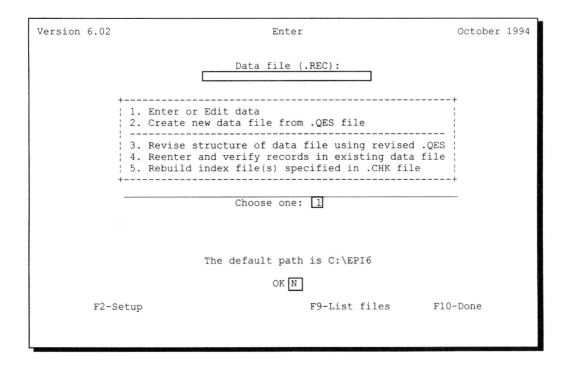

```
Version 6.02                      Enter                  October 1994


                        Data file (.REC):
                   +----------------------------+


      +---------------------------------------------------------+
      | 1. Enter or Edit data                                   |
      | 2. Create new data file from .QES file                  |
      | ------------------------------------------------------- |
      | 3. Revise structure of data file using revised .QES     |
      | 4. Reenter and verify records in existing data file     |
      | 5. Rebuild index file(s) specified in .CHK file         |
      +---------------------------------------------------------+

      _____
                        Choose one:  [1]



                    The default path is C:\EPI6

                          OK [N]

          F2-Setup                      F9-List files      F10-Done
```

Figure 4.3   The Enter screen.

Carry out the following sequence of commands to enter the data into the pat_data questionnaire file. First we select the 'questionnaire' file pat_data.qes.

- in the Data file (.REC): box type **pat_data** and press **Enter**
- in the 'Choose one:' box type **2** and press **Enter**. A new box appears on the screen 'New questionnaire file (.QES):'. Type **pat_data** and press **Enter**
- type **Y** in the **OK** box and press **Enter**.

A new screen appears with the three fields **gender**, **age** and **bloodgp** with spaces to type data in alongside:

- type in the first patient's data, i.e. 1, 21, 1, pressing Enter after each one
- type Y to write the data to disc.

Enter the data for the remaining nine patients as shown in Table 4.1. Press <F10> when all the data are entered. The data are ready to be analysed. Examples of analysis using this and other data are shown in the next three sections.

Help

Epi Info provides a comprehensive 'on-line' manual. This can be accessed via the main screen (Figure 4.1) by selecting the **Manual** menu. Select the **Contents** option which is highlighted by pressing Enter. The Contents page of the manual is shown in Figure 4.4.

```
Programs  Tutorials  Examples  Manual  File  Edit  Setup
+-[_]---------------------- C:\EPI6\EPI6CON.HLP ----------------------
                              Contents
¦¦ Print Table of Contents _____3_
¦
¦ Introduction:
¦
¦   Chapter 1    How To Use This Manual _____7_
¦
¦   Chapter 2    What Is Epi Info, Version 6? _____11_
¦
¦   Chapter 3    What's New in Version 6? _____17_
¦
¦   Chapter 4    Installing Epi Info _____35_
¦
¦   Chapter 5    Running Epi Info _____45_
¦
¦ Level I: Word Processing Functions
¦
¦   Chapter 6    Using EPED, the Epidemiologist's Editor, As a
¦                General Word Processor _____51_
¦
¦ F1-Help  F2-New  F3-Open  F4-Close  F5-Print  F8-Menu  F9-Save  F10-Quit
```

Figure 4.4   Contents page of the on-line Epi Info Manual.

Use the downward arrow key to browse through the Chapters and select any one by pressing the Enter key. Press <F10> to quit the Chapter when done. Press <F10> to exit the Manual.

A second option is to work through the 'on-line' tutorial exercises. From the main screen select the Tutorials menu and select a task from the list presented.

Help is also available as you work through tasks in Epi Info. Press <F1> to access it.

Exit

At any time in your work you may want to exit from Epi Info. To do this you must press <F10> from the main Epi Info screen (Figure 4.1).

Summary

This section has introduced you to Epi Info and has covered the first steps in using the package to analyse your data. This has included entering and saving data and using the online manual. It has also provided definitions of some of the key terminology used when analysing data. The following sections build on this work and introduce you to further features of the package.

Summarising and presenting data

The first step in any statistical analysis is summarising and presenting data. A simple summary statistic or graph will give you an immediate impression of the data you have collected. They also give a valuable check on any erroneous data that may have been entered by mistake and any missing data points.

Before we consider some methods used for summarising and presenting data, we need to consider the different types of data. These are nominal, ordinal, and interval and ratio data.

Nominal data: the observations are classified into categories that are different in character and cannot be measured or ordered. For example, gender, hair colour, blood group.

Ordinal data: the observations are classified into categories that can be ordered in an ascending series. For example, severity of an illness may be categorised as mild, moderate or severe.

Interval and ratio data: the observations are scores on a scale where the difference between scores is numerically equal. For example, height, weight.

The different types of data are important when considering the statistical analysis. The type of data determines the type of statistic that is appropriate for analysis. For a further discussion of this topic refer to Chapter 1 *An introduction to using statistics*.

Summarising data

Summary statistics include: the measures of location, for example mean, mode and median; and the measures of dispersion, for example range, interquartile range and standard deviation.

Summary statistics: measures of location

These give an idea of the position of an 'average' value on a particular scale of measurement.

The *mean* is the sum of all data points (observations or cases) divided by the number of data points, for example 7, 3, 11, 12, 9, 14, then the mean is $56/6 = 9.3$.

The *median* is the middle value of a set of observations ranked in order (or the average of the two central numbers when there is an even number of observations), for example 14, 9, 17, 21, 7, 18, 16, 22. When ranked in order of size these are 7, 9, 14, 16, 17, 18, 21, 22. There are eight scores, so the median is the average of the fourth and fifth scores: $(16+17)/2 = 16.5$.

By obtaining the median you know that half of the observations have values that are smaller than the median, and the other half have values larger than the median. You can find values that split the sample in other ways. For example, you can find the value below which fall 25% of the data values. Such values are called 'percentiles', since they tell you the percentage of cases with values below and above them. For example, 25% of cases will have values smaller than the 25th percentile and 75% of cases will have values larger than the 25th percentile. The median is known as the 50th percentile, since 50% of cases have values less than the median and 50% have values greater than the median.

The *mode* is the most common value of a set of observations, for example 5, 2, 3, 4, 5, 6, 5, then the mode is 5.

Summary statistics: measures of dispersion

These are ways of describing the variability of data and include the range, interquartile range and standard deviation.

The **range** is the difference between the largest and smallest observations, for example 19, 21, 22, 22, 25, 27, 28, 42, then the range is $42 - 19 = 23$. A large value for the range tells you that the largest and smallest values differ substantially. It doesn't tell you about the variability of the values between the smallest and largest. A better measure of variability is the **interquartile range**. This is the difference between the 75th and 25th percentile values (see above).

One of the most commonly used measures of variability is called the **standard deviation**. It indicates the extent to which the scores (values) deviate from the mean score. It is defined as the average deviation from the mean.

Table 4.2   Frequency table of blood groups

Group	No. of patients
O	56
A	31
B	18
AB	15
Total	**120**

Presenting data

Data presentation techniques include: bar charts, histograms, and frequency tables.

Data presentation: frequency table

A frequency table is a simple and effective way of presenting data. It is particularly suitable when observations fall into one of a number of different categories (nominal data). An example is shown below in Table 4.2.

The first column shows the possible categories that the observations could take and the second column shows the frequency with which each category occurs. This is known as a 'frequency distribution'.

Data presentation: bar chart

A bar chart displays the frequency count for each category of a frequency distribution. Figure 4.5 shows the number of patients in each of the blood groups.

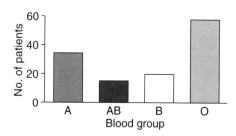

Figure 4.5   Bar chart of blood groups.

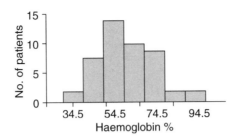

Figure 4.6   Histogram of haemoglobin %.

Data presentation: histogram

Histograms are similar to bar charts except that each bar represents a range of values. For example a single bar may represent all the patients in Figure 4.3 with a haemoglobin percentage between 30 and 39. The midpoint, i.e. 34.5, is used to label the bar. A histogram of the haemoglobin data is shown in Figure 4.6.

Table 4.3   Haemoglobin data

Haemoglobin %	Frequency (no. of patients)
30–39	2
40–49	7
50–59	14
60–69	10
70–79	8
80–89	2
90–99	2

Table 4.3 shows the number of patients with various percentage haemoglobin counts.

Exercise 1

This exercise explains how to summarise and present data using Epi Info. The file created in the first section **pat_data.rec** is used to demonstrate the main features of the package.

From the **Programs menu** select **ANALYSIS of data**. At the EPI6> prompt type: **Read pat_data** and press **Enter**. Type **list** and press **Enter** to view the data.

1.   Generate summary statistics for **age**:
     *   type **means age /n** and press **Enter**
     *   view the output (ignore the line on the Student's t-Test):

```
Dataset:   C:\EPI6\PAT_DATA.REC (10 records)            Free memory: 266K
Criteria: All records selected                          Time:    0.00 sec
+--------------------------- Output - Screen ----------------------------+
|                                                                        |
|=========> means age /n                                                 |
|                                                                        |
|                                                                        |
|AGE                                                                     |
|                                                                        |
|        Total          Sum        Mean    Variance    Std Dev    Std Err |
|           10          420      42.000     262.222     16.193      5.121 |
|                                                                        |
|      Minimum       25%ile      Median      75%ile    Maximum       Mode |
|       19.000       26.000      42.000      55.000     65.000     19.000 |
|                                                                        |
|Student's "t", testing whether mean differs from zero.                  |
|T statistic = 8.202,  df =      9   p-value = 0.00010                    |
|                                                                        |
|                                                                        |
|--------------------------- Commands -----------------------------------|
|EPI6>                                                               |    |
|EPI6> means age /n                                                      |
|EPI6>                                                                   |
| F1-Help  F2-Commands  F3-Variables  F4-Browse  F5-Printer on  F9-DOS  F10-Quit
```

2.   Generate a frequency table for **bloodgp**:
  - type **freq bloodgp** and press **Enter**
  - view the output:

```
Dataset:   C:\EPI6\PAT_DATA.REC (10 records)            Free memory: 265K
Criteria: All records selected                          Time:    0.00 sec
+--------------------------- Output - Screen ----------------------------+
|                                                                        |
|BLOODGP |  Freq  Percent    Cum.                                        |
|--------+---------------------                                          |
| 1      |     3   30.0%     30.0%                                       |
| 2      |     1   10.0%     40.0%                                       |
| 3      |     2   20.0%     60.0%                                       |
| 4      |     4   40.0%    100.0%                                       |
|--------+---------------------                                          |
|  Total |    10  100.0%                                                 |
|                                                                        |
|        Total          Sum        Mean    Variance    Std Dev    Std Err |
|           10           27       2.700       1.789      1.337      0.423 |
|                                                                        |
|      Minimum       25%ile      Median      75%ile    Maximum       Mode |
|<more>                                                                  |
|--------------------------- Commands -----------------------------------|
```

3. Generate a bar chart for **bloodgp**:
    *   type **bar bloodgp** and press **Enter**
    *   examine the output (press the space bar when done).
4. Generate a histogram for **age**:
    *   type **histogram age** and press **Enter**
    *   examine the output (press the space bar when done).

Testing hypotheses

Introduction

One of the most important aspects of statistics is that concerned with making inferences or generalisations about a particular population on the basis of a sample drawn from that population. An assumption about the population is called a 'statistical hypothesis'.

The hypothesis we are trying to test is called the 'null' hypothesis (denoted H_0). The null hypothesis is the frame of reference against which you will judge your sample results. A contrary assumption is called the 'alternative' hypothesis (denoted H_1); this claims that the results differ from the frame of reference in a real or significant manner.

Hypotheses are best described by examples. Suppose we have a new drug to treat depression, drug x, and we want to discover whether it is more effective than an existing drug, drug y. The simplest hypothesis to test is that there is no difference in effectiveness between drug x and drug y. This would be the null hypothesis; it postulates the state of no difference. The alternative hypothesis would be that there is a difference in effectiveness between the two drugs.

We use appropriate experimental methods to gather evidence and then try to decide whether or not the null hypothesis is likely to be true. If the evidence is inconsistent with the null hypothesis then it is 'rejected'. If the evidence from the sample is consistent with the hypothesis then it is 'accepted'. The procedure we adopt in investigating the evidence is a 'statistical test'.

The result of a test is a decision to choose either H_0 or H_1. Such a decision is subject to uncertainty or error. Because of this the result is expressed as a probability (the p value).

There are numerous statistical tests available for analysing the significance of data. The selection of the appropriate test depends on the nature of the data to be analysed.

Two broad categories of tests have been developed and are referred to as 'parametric' and 'non-parametric' tests. Parametric tests are generally considered to be more powerful than non-parametric tests because they take into account more information about differences in scores. In general, parametric tests should only be used if your data fit the following specifications:

*   interval or ratio data
*   scores are normally distributed
*   the two sets of scores have the same variance.

A detailed examination of these points is beyond the scope of this chapter. Interested readers can refer to statistics textbooks in *Further reading and resources* on p. 101. Below, however, are some of the major tests, with a brief description of the appropriate data for each one. In each case analysis of the data is shown using Epi Info. The data sets are examples only; they are used simply to demonstrate the different features of the statistical software.

Parametric tests

Paired t-Test

The paired-samples t-Test is used to test if two related samples come from populations with the same mean. The related, or paired, samples often result from an experiment in which the same person is observed before and after an intervention.

Example: To investigate the effects of exercise on blood glucose level in diabetics, blood glucose concentration (mmol/l) was measured in patients before and after a period of exercise (Table 4.4).

Exercise 2

This exercise explains how to use Epi Info to analyse paired data using the t-Test. The data set for the analysis is the blood glucose measurements.

First we need to enter the data. Create a new QES file following the methods presented previously. Create two fields named **before** and **after**, each of type ## (number) with three digits before the decimal point and with two decimal places. Save the file as **diabet.qes**. Enter the data for each patient shown in Table 4.4 via the **Enter** program. Press **<F10>** when done. Select **ANALYSIS of data** from the main menu.

1. Type **read diabet**, to load the file.
2. Type **define diff ###.##**, to create a new field (required for the analysis). Press **Enter**.

Table 4.4   Blood glucose data

Patient	Blood glucose before	Blood glucose after
1	15.3	9.2
2	16.7	10.3
3	17.0	8.8
4	14.2	12.3
5	16.5	11.0
6	17.9	8.8
7	16.3	8.4
8	17.3	9.9
9	15.8	10.3

3. Type **diff = before – after**, to calculate the difference between the scores for each subject.
4. Type **freq diff**, to obtain the t statistic and p value. Examine the output.

```
Dataset:  C:\EPI6\DIABET.REC (9 records)              Free memory: 267K
Criteria: All records selected                        Time:   0.00 sec
+------------------------ Output - Screen -------------------------+
|   7.90 |    1   11.1%    77.8%                                    |
|   8.20 |    1   11.1%    88.9%                                    |
|   9.10 |    1   11.1%   100.0%                                    |
| -------+---------------------                                    |
|  Total |    9  100.0%                                            |
|                                                                  |
|       Total        Sum       Mean   Variance   Std Dev   Std Err |
|           9         58      6.444      4.465     2.113     0.704  |
|                                                                  |
|     Minimum     25%ile     Median     75%ile   Maximum      Mode |
|       1.900      5.500      6.400      7.900     9.100     5.500  |
|                                                                  |
|Student's "t", testing whether mean differs from zero.            |
|T statistic = 9.149,  df =      8    p-value = 0.00010            |
|                                                                  |
|------------------------------- Commands -------------------------|
|EPI6> diff = before - after                                       |
|EPI6> freq diff                                                   |
```

The test statistic t has a value of –9.149 and p = 0.00010 (2-Tail Sig).

Independent-samples t-Test

The independent-samples t-Test is used when two samples of subjects provide scores on a measure. The t-Test compares the means of the two samples.

In a trial of zinc sulphate on wound healing, nine patients were given oral zinc therapy in addition to normal treatment. A further nine patients received only their normal treatment. The time taken for 'complete healing' (in days) was measured; the data are shown in Table 4.5.

Table 4.5   Zinc sulphate data

Normal treatment and zinc sulphate	Normal treatment only
33	40
34	63
52	57
46	45
45	34
69	26
47	45
51	56
44	73

Exercise 3

This exercise explains how to use Epi Info to analyse independent-samples data using the t-Test. The data set for the analysis is the zinc sulphate data.

First we need to enter the data. Create a new QES file following the methods presented previously. Create two fields named **healtime** and **group**, each of type ## (number) with two digits before the decimal point and with 0 decimal places. Save the file as **wound.qes.** Enter the data for each patient shown in Table 4.5 via the **Enter** program; the first nine values of healtime (left-hand column of above table) with group = 1 and the second nine values of healtime with group = 2. Press **<F10>** when done. Select **ANALYSIS of data** from the main menu.

1. Type **read wound**, to load the file.
2. Type **means healtime group**, to calculate the test statistic. Examine the output.

```
Dataset:  C:\EPI6\WOUND.REC (18 records)              Free memory: 262K
Criteria: All records selected
+--------------------------- Output - Screen ----------------------------+
     Total |    9     9 |    18

 GROUP             Obs       Total       Mean    Variance    Std Dev
 1                   9         421     46.778     112.944     10.628
 2                   9         439     48.778     218.944     14.797
 Difference                             -2.000

 GROUP         Minimum     25%ile      Median      75%ile     Maximum        Mode
 1              33.000     44.000      46.000      51.000      69.000      33.000
 2              26.000     40.000      45.000      57.000      73.000      45.000

                               ANOVA
                (For normally distributed data only)

 Variation          SS    df          MS   F statistic    p-value    t-value
 Between        18.000     1      18.000         0.108    0.744474   0.329348
 ------------------------------ Commands --------------------------------
 EPI6> means healtime group
 EPI6>
 EPI6>
 F1-Help  F2-Commands  F3-Variables  F4-Browse  F5-Printer on  F9-DOS  F10-Quit
```

The test statistic t = –0.329 and p = 0.744 (2-Tail Sig).

Non-parametric tests

Wilcoxon Matched-Pairs Test

This is the non-parametric counterpart of the related samples t-Test. Unfortunately the Wilcoxon Matched-Pairs Signed-Ranks Test is not available in Epi Info.

Table 4.6   **Energy expenditure data**

Energy expenditure (MJ/day)	
Lean (N = 13)	**Obese (N = 9)**
6.13	8.79
7.05	9.19
7.48	9.21
7.48	9.68
7.53	9.69
7.58	9.97
7.90	11.51
8.08	11.85
8.09	12.79
8.11	
8.40	
10.15	
10.88	

Mann-Whitney U Test

This is the non-parametric counterpart of the independent-samples t-Test.

Example: The energy expenditure of lean and obese groups of female subjects were measured over a 24-hour period (Table 4.6).

Exercise 4

This exercise explains how to use Epi Info to analyse independent-samples data using the Mann-Whitney U Test. The data set for the analysis is the energy expenditure data shown in Table 4.6.

First we need to enter the data. Create a new QES file following the methods presented previously. Create two fields named **energy** and **group**. **Energy** of type ## (number) with two digits before the decimal point and with two decimal places, and **group** of type ## with one digit before the decimal point and with 0 decimal places. Save the file as **energy.qes.** Enter the data for each patient via the **Enter** program; the 13 values of energy expenditure (left-hand column of above table) with group = 1 and the other nine values with group = 2. Press **<F10>** when done. Select **ANALYSIS of data** from the main menu.

1. Type **read energy**, to load the file.
2. Type **means energy group**, to calculate the test statistic. Examine the output.

```
Dataset:  C:\EPI6\ENERGY.REC (22 records)           Free memory: 264K
Criteria: All records selected                      Time:    0.00 sec
+-------------------------- Output - Screen --------------------------+
¦Between        26.485    1      26.485      15.567  0.001080  3.945565 ¦
¦Within         34.026   20       1.701                                ¦
¦Total          60.512   21                                            ¦
¦                                                                      ¦
¦                 Bartlett's test for homogeneity of variance          ¦
¦     Bartlett's chi square =   0.136  deg freedom = 1   p-value = 0.712048 ¦
¦                                                                      ¦
¦              The variances are homogeneous with 95% confidence.      ¦
¦       If samples are also normally distributed, ANOVA results can be used. ¦
¦                                                                      ¦
¦                                                                      ¦
¦Mann-Whitney or Wilcoxon Two-Sample Test (Kruskal-Wallis test for two groups) ¦
¦                                                                      ¦
¦Kruskal-Wallis H (equivalent to Chi square) =       9.648             ¦
¦                         Degrees of freedom =          1              ¦
¦                                p value =       0.001896              ¦
¦-------------------------------- Commands ----------------------------¦
¦EPI6> means energy group                                             ¦
```

The p value = 0.001896.

Contingency tables

The techniques introduced here involve data in the form of frequencies. In other words, they deal with the situation where we are counting the number of times a particular event occurs.

To determine whether an appointment reminder system is associated with a decrease in the number of non-attendance at a health-screening clinic. The results for a random sample of people are shown in Table 4.7.

This is called a contingency table. This type of data is suited to analysis with the Chi-Square Test (denoted χ^2). The null hypothesis is that the outcome, i.e. whether patients attended or did not attend their appointments, is independent of the reminder status.

Table 4.7   Attendance data

Status	Attended	Did not attend	Total
Reminder	30	9	39
No reminder	15	6	21
Total	45	15	60

Exercise 5

This exercise explains how to use Epi Info to analyse contingency table data using the Chi-Square Test. The data set for the analysis is the attendance data shown in Table 4.7.

Select **EPITABLE calculator** from the main menu. Select the **Compare** menu, then **Proportion**, then **r × c table**.

1.   Press the **Enter** key three times to accept a 2 × 2 table.
2.   Type **30**, then press the **Tab** key, followed by **9 Tab**, **15 Tab**, **6 Tab**.
3.   Press the **Enter** key to **Calculate**. Examine the output.

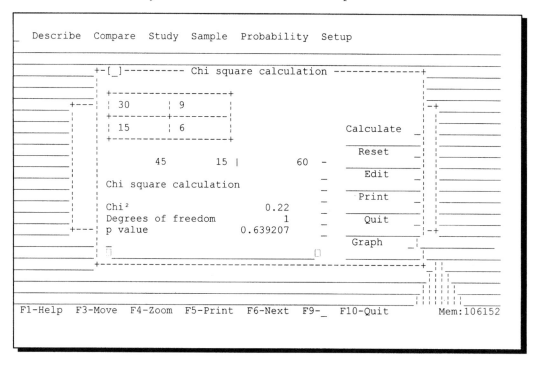

The test statistic is 0.22 and p = 0.639.

Examining relationships

This section considers the relationships between two measures. If two measures are shown to be related then (a) the description of the data can be simplified and (b) further research can be undertaken to determine the mechanisms which cause the measures to be related. The method of correlation is presented.

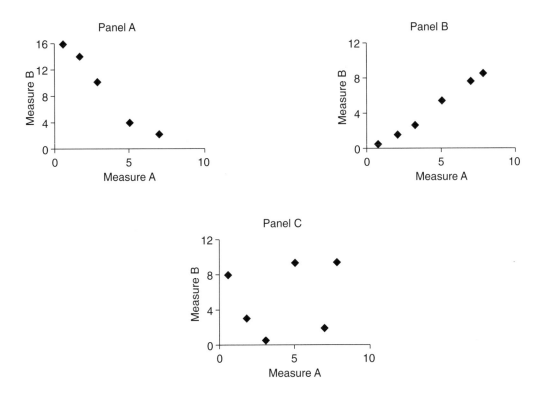

Figure 4.7   Associations of two measures.

Correlation

Correlation is a measure of the extent to which two measures, for example height and weight, are related. The statistical measure of relation (or association) is known as the 'correlation coefficient' (denoted by the symbol r). Its value lies between -1 and $+1$; a large negative r indicates a negative association (Figure 4.7, Panel A); a large positive r represents a positive association (Figure 4.7, Panel B); and a small r (either positive or negative) or $r = 0$ indicates little or no association at all (Figure 4.7, Panel C).

Example: Table 4.8 gives the results of a study in which 10 women had their haemoglobin level and packed cell volume (PCV) measured, together with their age.

Exercise 6

This exercise explains how to use Epi Info to analyse the relationship between two measures using correlation. The data set for the analysis is the haemoglobin and packed cell volume data shown in Table 4.8.

Table 4.8   Haemoglobin and packed cell volume data

Patient	Hb	PCV	Age
1	11.1	35	20
2	10.7	45	22
3	12.4	47	25
4	14.0	50	28
5	13.1	31	28
6	10.5	30	31
7	9.6	25	32
8	12.5	33	35
9	13.5	35	38
10	13.9	40	40

First we need to enter the data. Create a new QES file following the methods presented previously. Add two fields, named **Hb** (two digits before the decimal point and with one decimal place) and **PCV** (two digits, no decimal places). Save the file as **hb.qes.** Enter the data for each patient via the **Enter** program. Press **<F10>** when done. Select **ANALYSIS of data** from the main menu.

1.   Type **read hb**, to load the file.
2.   Type **scatter hb pcv** to give a scatter diagram.
3.   Type **regress hb pcv** to give the correlation coefficient. Examine the output.

```
Dataset:   C:\EPI6\HB.REC (10 records)                    Free memory: 267K
Criteria: All records selected                            Time:    0.05 sec
+---------------------------- Output - Screen ----------------------------+
|========> regress hb pcv                                                 |
|Correlation coefficient: r  = 0.48                                       |
|                         r^2= 0.23                                       |
|95% confidence limits:   -0.21 < R < 0.85                                |
|                                                                         |
|Source             df   Sum of Squares   Mean Square    F-statistic      |
|Regression          1          5.0241       5.0241          2.39         |
|Residuals           8         16.7969       2.0996                       |
|Total               9         21.8210                                    |
|                                                                         |
|ß Coefficients                                                           |
|                                                                         |
|                        ß            95% confidence            Partial   |
|Variable    Mean    coefficient    Lower     Upper    Std Error  F-test  |
|PCV       37.1000    0.0918978   -0.024543  0.208338  0.059408  2.3928   |
|Y-Intercept          8.7205917                                           |
|                                                                         |
|---------------------------- Commands -----------------------------------|
|EPI6> scatter hb pcv                                                     |
|EPI6> regress hb pcv                                                     |
|EPI6>                                                                    |
| F1-Help  F2-Commands  F3-Variables  F4-Browse  F5-Printer on  F9-DOS  F10-Quit |
```

The correlation coefficient, $r = 0.48$.

Summary

This chapter has provided an introduction to the statistics package Epi Info. Introductory material was presented in the first section, which included a step-by-step guide to entering data into the package. This was followed by three key sections, which described how to use Epi Info to summarise and analyse different types of data sets. In each section, several illustrative examples were presented together with screen shots from the package showing expected outputs.

The chapter was written with the beginner in mind and to encourage use of the package rather than to produce an expert user. However, after working through the chapter it is likely that you have more questions now than when you started. Fortunately help is at hand from a number of sources. First, Epi Info contains a comprehensive on-line user manual which should always be consulted should a question arise. Second, other manuals and textbooks are available, examples of which are listed in *Further reading* (below). Finally, there are many experienced users of Epi Info in the field of health services research who may be willing and able to help.

When using a statistical package to analyse data we should not forget the wider context of the research process. This includes an appreciation of the research design, data collection, data analysis and interpretation of results. These aspects have not been discussed at length in this chapter. Further information can be found in other Trent Focus volumes in this series and textbooks of statistics, again examples of which are listed in *Further reading* (below).

This chapter has provided a practical step-by-step guide to Epi Info for those new to the package. It is hoped that it has provided you with a firm foundation and confidence in using Epi Info.

Further reading and resources

Altman D G (1991) *Practical Statistics for Medical Research*. Chapman and Hall, London.

Bland M (1995) *An Introduction to Medical Statistics*. Oxford University Press, Oxford.

Brown R A and Swanson Beck J (1994) *Medical Statistics on Computers*. BMJ Publishing Group, London.

Puri B K (1996) *Statistics for the Health Sciences using SPSS*. Saunders, London.

Rowntree D (1991) *Statistics without Tears*. Penguin, London.

Swinscow T D V (1996) *Statistics at Square One* (9e) (revised by M J Campbell). BMJ Publishing Group, London.

Epi Info can be downloaded and used without charge from the World Wide Web at: http://www.cdc.gov/epo/epi/epiinfo.htm

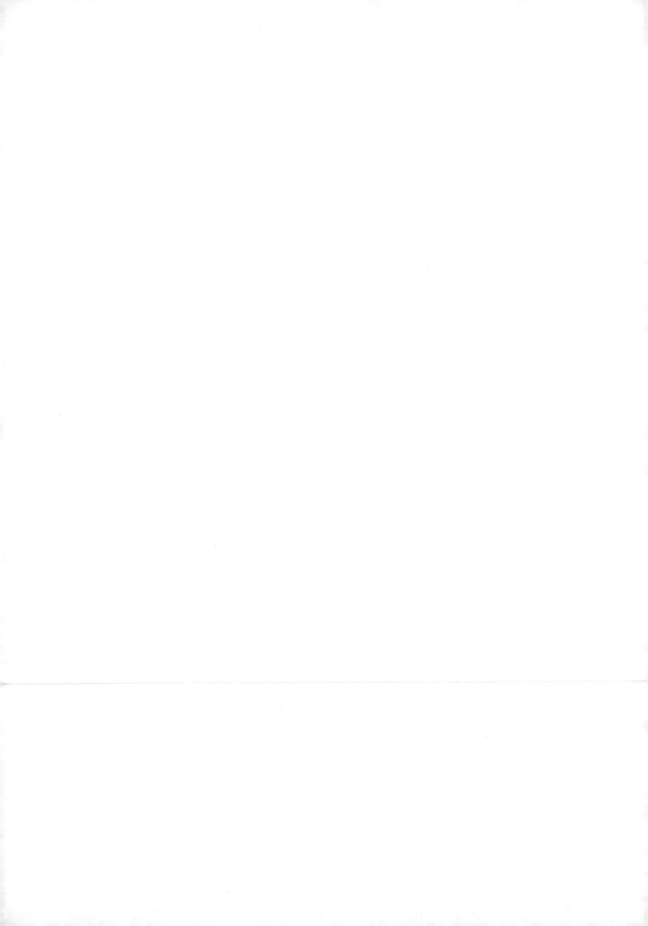

Glossary

ANOVA (Analysis of Variance)
a test of statistical significance for assessing the difference between two or more sample means. Also known as the F-Test.

Bias
a derivation of the results from the truth. This can either be due to random error or, more likely, due to systematic error. The latter could be caused by, for example, sampling or poor questionnaire design.

Chi-Square (χ^2) Test
a non-parametric test (q.v.) of statistical significance. It is usually applied to cross-tabulated nominal data. It is used as a measure of association between two nominal variables.

Confidence interval
the range of values around a mean or point for a specific variable. The confidence intervals are specified by plus or minus two standard deviations either side of the mean or point, with a 95% likelihood that the true value lies within this range.

Control group
the group in an experiment which is not exposed to the intervention or independent variable. The control group exists to provide a baseline comparison for the intervention group so as to measure the influence of the independent variable.

Correlation
the degree to which two variables change together. A correlation may be linear or curvilinear. They may be positive or negative (also known as inverse correlations).

Descriptive design
one which seeks to describe the distribution of variables for a particular topic. Descriptive studies can be quantitative, i.e. a survey, but they do not involve the use of a deliberate intervention. However, it is possible to carry out correlational analysis of the existing variables in a descriptive study.

Descriptive statistics
used to describe and summarise variables within a data set, including describing relationships between variables. They do not seek to generalise the findings from the sample to the wider population, unlike inferential statistics.

Effect size
the magnitude of difference between two or more groups. For example in a drug trial comparing a novel drug with

	an existing one, the difference (proportion or percentage) in efficacy of the two drugs is known as the effect size.
Error	can be due to two sources: random error and systematic error. Random error is due to chance, whilst systematic error is due to an identifiable source, such as sampling bias or response bias.
Experimental design	one in which there is direct control over the use of an intervention. In a classic experimental design, the subjects are randomised into intervention and control group and the dependent variable is assessed before and after treatment. See also RCT.
External validity	relates to the extent to which the findings from a study can be generalised (from the sample) to a wider population (and be claimed to be representative).
Hypothesis	statement about the relationship between the dependent and the independent variables to be studied. Traditionally the null hypothesis is assumed to be correct, until research demonstrates that the null hypothesis is incorrect. See also Null hypothesis.
Incidence	can be defined as the number of new spells of a phenomenon, e.g. illness, in a defined population in a specified period. An incidence rate would be the rate at which new cases of the phenomena occur in a given population. See also Prevalence.
Independent variable	is one which 'causes' the dependent variable. The independent variable takes the form of the intervention or treatment in an experiment and is manipulated to demonstrate change in the dependent variable.
Inferential statistics	are those class of statistics which are used to make generalisations from a sample to a population.
Internal validity	relates to the validity of the study itself, including both the design and the instruments used.
Intervention	the independent variable in an experimental design. An intervention could take the form of treatment, such as drug treatment. Those subjects selected to receive the intervention in an experiment are placed in the 'intervention' group.
Mean	arithmetic average of scores in a distribution of values.

Median
a measure of central tendency. It is the mid-point or middle value where all the values are placed in order. It is less susceptible to distortion by extreme values than the mean, and is a suitable descriptive statistic for both ordinal and interval data.

Mode
a measure of central tendency. It is the most frequently occurring or most common value in a set of observations. It can be used for any measurement level, but is most suited for describing nominal or categorical data.

Nominal data
also known as categorical data, is a set of unordered categories. Each category is represented by a different numerical code, but the codes or numbers are allocated on an arbitrary basis and have no numerical meaning. See also Ordinal data.

Non-parametric

statistics
unlike parametric statistics, do not make any assumptions about the underlying distribution of data. Non-parametric statistics are therefore suitable for skewed data and nominal and ordinal levels of measurement.

Normal distribution
A frequency distribution whose graphic representation has a symmetric, bell-shaped form in which most values congregate around the mean, median and mode. Its characteristics are often referred to when deciding upon which type of statistical test to use.

Null hypothesis
is a hypothesis that states there is no relationship between the variables being studied. The null hypothesis is assumed to be correct until research demonstrates that it is incorrect. This process is known as falsification.

Ordinal data
is composed of a set of categories which can be placed in an order. Each category is represented by a numeric code which in turn represents the same order as the data. However, the numbers do not represent the distance between each category. For instance, a variable describing patient satisfaction may be coded as follows: dissatisfied 1, neither 2, satisfied 3. The code 2 *cannot* be interpreted as being twice that of code 1.

Panel study
is another term for a longitudinal or cohort study, where individuals are interviewed repeatedly over a period of time.

Parallel design   refers to the traditional experimental design where the intervention group and the control group are run alongside each other. An alternative to a parallel design is a crossover design.

Parametric tests   require data to be at interval level, derived from normal distributions and for there to be a similarity of spread between samples, known as 'homogeneity of variance'. Consequently, these tests are seen as more powerful than their non-parametric equivalents.

Placebo   usually an inert drug or 'sugar-coated pill' used to simulate drug treatment in a control group in an experimental design. *Placebo* is Latin for 'I will please'.

Population   a term used in research which refers to <u>all</u> the potential subjects or units of interest who share the same characteristics which would make them eligible for entry into a study. The population of potential subjects is also known as the 'sampling frame'.

Power   the probability of showing a difference between groups when there is a real difference between the groups, and therefore reducing the chance of committing a Type II error. Power calculations are used to find out how likely we are to detect an effect for a given sample size, effect size, and level of significance. Power is usually denoted as $1-\beta$. The minimum recommended power level is 80%.

Prevalence   the number of cases as subjects with a given condition or disease within a specified time period. The prevalence of a condition would include all those people with the condition even if the condition started prior to the start of the specified time period. See also Incidence.

Prospective study   one that is planned from the beginning and takes a forward-looking approach. Subjects are followed over time and interventions can be introduced as appropriate.

Qualitative   research usually deals with the human experience and is based on analysis of words rather than numbers. Qualitative research methods seek to explore rich information usually collected from a fairly small sample and includes methods such as in-depth interviews, focus groups, action research and ethnographic studies.

Quantitative	research is essentially concerned with numerical measurement and numerical data. All experimental research is based on a quantitative approach. Quantitative research tends to be based on larger sample sizes in order to produce results which can be generalised to a wider population.
Quasi-experimental design	one in which the researcher has no control over who receives the intervention and who does not. An alternative to randomisation as used in experimental research, is the process of matching.
Quota sample	a form of non-random sampling and one that is commonly used in market research. The sample is designed to meet certain quotas, set usually to obtain certain numbers by age, sex and social class. The sample selected within each quota is selected by convenience, rather than random methods.
Random error	non-systematic bias which can negate the influence of the independent variable. Reliability is affected by random error.
Randomisation	the random assignment of subjects to intervention and control groups. Randomisation is a way of ensuring that chance dictates who receives which treatment. In this way all extraneous variables should be provided for. Random allocation does not mean haphazard allocation.
Randomised control trial (RCT)	seen as the 'gold standard' of experimental design. As the name implies, subjects are randomly allocated to either the intervention or the control group.
Ratio level data	similar to interval data in that there is an equal distance between each value except that ratio data does possess a true zero. An example of ratio data would be age.
Reliability	concerned with the extent to which a measure gives consistent results. It is also a pre-condition for validity.
Representativeness	the extent to which a sample of subjects is representative of the wider population. If a sample is not representative, then the findings may not be generalisable.
Response rate	the proportion of people who have participated in a study or completed a question. It is calculated by dividing the total number of people who have participated by those who were approached or asked to participate.

Sample   subset of a population selected by the researcher. A random sample is one attempt to ensure that each member of a population has an equal chance of being picked.

Sampling frame   the pool of potential subjects which share a similar criteria for entry into a study. The sampling frame is also known as the 'population'.

Significance level   usually stated as the *p* value. A significance level is commonly set at either 0.01 (a one in 100 chance of being incorrect) or 0.05 (a one in 20 chance of being incorrect).

Significance tests   may be parametric or non-parametric. A significance test is used to detect statistically significant differences between groups or associations between variables.

Snowballing   a non-probability method of sampling commonly employed in qualitative research. Recruited subjects nominate other potential subjects for inclusion in the study.

Spurious correlation   an apparent correlation between two variables when there is no causal link between them. Spurious relationships are often accounted for a third confounding variable. Once this third variable is controlled, the correlation between the two variables disappears.

Standard deviation   a summary measure of dispersion. It is a summary of how closely clustered or dispersed are the values around the mean. For data that is normally distributed, 68% of all cases lie within one standard deviation either side of the mean and 95% of all cases are within two standard deviations either side of the mean.

Standard error   the standard deviation of the estimate.

Statistical Package for the Social Sciences (SPSS)   is an increasingly popular and easy-to-use software package for data analysis.

Statistical significance   the numerical likelihood or probability that the result or one more extreme has occurred by chance.

Statistics   the analysis of numerical data about samples of populations.

Stratified sample   one where the sample is divided into a number of different strata based on certain criteria such as age, sex or ethnic group. The sample selection within each strata, however, is based on a random or probability method. A stratified sample is a way of ensuring that the sample is representative rather than leaving it to chance.

Survey

a method of collecting large-scale quantitative data, but does not use an experimental design. With a survey there is no control over who receives the intervention or when. Instead a survey design can examine the real world and describe existing relationships. A survey can be either simply descriptive or a correlation.

Theoretical sampling

a sampling method used in qualitative research, whereby the sample is selected on the basis of the theory and the needs of the emerging theory. It does not seek to be representative.

t-Test

a test of statistical significance for assessing the difference between two sample means. It can only be used if the data distribution follows a normal distribution and if the two sets of data have similar variations.

Type I error

is the error of falsely rejecting a true null hypothesis and thereby accepting that there is a statistical difference when one does not exist. The chance of committing a Type I error is known as alpha (α) and is expressed as a p value.

Type I error

is the error of falsely rejecting a true null hypothesis and thereby accepting that there is a statistical difference when one does not exist. The chance of committing a Type I error is known as alpha (α).

Type II error

the error of failing to reject a false null hypothesis or wrongly accepting a false null hypothesis. The likelihood of committing a Type II error is known as beta (β). The conventional level of statistical power ($1-\beta$) is usually set at 80% or 0.8.

Validity

the extent to which a study measures what it purports to measure. There are many different types of validity.

Variable

an indicator of a concept. It is a phenomenon which varies and must be measurable. An outcome variable is known as the dependent variable and the effect variable is known as the independent variable. The independent variable has a causal effect on the dependent variable.

Weighting   a correction factor which is applied to data in the analysis
                             phase to make the sample representative. For instance, if a
                             disproportionate stratified sampling technique has been
                             used, then the total data may need to be reweighted to
                             make it representative of the total population. Weighting is
                             also used to correct for non-response, when the respondents
                             are known to be biased in a systematic way.

Index